Dawn A. Marcus, MD · Philip A. Bain, MD

Effective Migraine Treatment in Pregnant and Lactating Women: A Practical Guide

Foreword by Donna Shoupe, MD

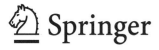 Springer

Dawn A. Marcus, MD
Professor Department
    of Anesthesiology
University of Pittsburgh
Pittsburgh, PA
USA

Philip A. Bain, MD
Dean Health System
Madison, WI
USA

ISBN 978-1-60327-438-8   e-ISBN 978-1-60327-439-5
DOI 10.1007/978-1-60327-439-5

Library of Congress Control Number: 2008942074

"A wonderful, practical resource that supplies much-needed expert information on a common pregnancy problem."
– Elizabeth W. Loder, MD, Chief of the Division of Headache and Pain, John R. Graham Headache Center

The book *Effective Migraine Treatment in Pregnant and Lactating Women: A Practical Guide* is a much needed first of its kind, dealing with pregnancy and lactation for women with migraine. Designed for busy practitioners, each chapter begins with key points and a case study and ends with Practical Pointers that succinctly summarize key messages. Throughout the chapters are relevant "Pearls for the Practitioner." In addition, there are examples of education to present to patients, treatment and medication algorithms, and other downloadable (from the CD-ROM version of the book) information for clinicians. This book is truly a masterpiece and provides insightful information for all healthcare professionals who manage women with migraine.
–Roger K. Cady, MD, Medical Director of the Headache Care Center in the Primary Care Network

Foreword

Effective Migraine Treatment in Pregnant and the Lactating Women: A Practical Guide provides a comprehensive review of the pathophysiology, activating factors, course, frequency, work-up, treatment and follow-up of migraine headaches in pregnant and lactating women. This text reviews the vast and diverse treatment options now available including medications, life-style modifications, stress management, complementary medicine, exercise, diet and nutritional therapies. Considering that women are more than twice as likely to experience migraines as men and 1 in 5 women will experience migraines during her reproductive years, this book is appreciated as a valuable resource.

Effective Migraine Treatment in Pregnant and the Lactating Women: A Practical Guide provides headache diaries, patient educational tools, as well as detailed instructions for pain management, use of rescue medications, physical therapy exercises and preconception counseling. Readers will develop a practical and extended approach to the evaluation and treatment of the pregnant and lactating headache sufferers. In all, this book is an excellent resource for healthcare providers taking care of pregnant or breastfeeding women suffering with migraines as well as providers treating reproductive aged women with migraines that are anticipating pregnancy.

Obstetrician/gynecologist   Donna Shoupe, MD
Los Angeles, CA

Preface

Migraine affects nearly one in every five adult women, with the peak prevalence during the mid-thirties. Since women are typically affected with migraine during their reproductive years, it is not surprising that many women in their childbearing years will seek medical care for migraine during pregnancy and lactation. Clinicians are often apprehensive about treating migraines in fertile and pregnant women because of concerns about treatment effects on their unborn babies, often resulting in under-treatment of disabling pain and nausea. Fortunately, a variety of relatively safe and effective drug and non-drug treatments are available for migraine-related pain and nausea during conception, pregnancy, and nursing. This book provides a comprehensive resource to address diagnosis, testing, and treatment of headaches in reproductively fertile women.

The term *safe* is used in this book to describe treatments that are considered to be relatively safe for women to use during pregnancy or when nursing. Clinicians using this information should remember that all drugs have certain risks of adverse events and relative safety is often based on limited data, particularly during pregnancy. Ideally, the treatment of headaches in pregnant or lactating women would not need to include medications; however, this is not always feasible. Relative safety needs to be balanced against the consequences of untreated headache, which might include vomiting, dehydration, and disability. Recommendations in this book are based on published evidence in the literature and clinical experience, with full referencing for suggested therapies.

Dr. Dawn Marcus is a neurologist who has devoted a large portion of her professional career to the treatment of patients with chronic pain and headache. She developed a successful multidisciplinary headache clinic at the University of Pittsburgh Medical Center and currently directs headache research there. Her years of clinical experience resulted in developing practical tips and resources for managing difficult headache populations. She is an active writer and lecturer on topics related to headache and chronic pain and has authored several practical books for both healthcare providers and a lay audience (www.dawnmarcusmd.com).

Dr. Philip Bain is a practicing internist in a large multispecialty organization in Madison, WI. Though he has a large general internal medicine practice, he has had a long-standing interest in the diagnosis and treatment of headache disorders by primary care providers. He has developed a myriad of helpful patient handouts and primary care tools that have helped primary care providers treat headache patients efficiently and consistently. His focus on office workflow has resulted in the development of a variety of practical tools to assist clinicians in treating pregnant and nursing migraine sufferers both efficiently and effectively.

Together Drs. Marcus and Bain bring a wealth of practical, ready-to-use, clinically tested tips and recommendations to treat women with headaches during pregnancy and nursing. This book uniquely answers frequently asked questions by patients and provides healthcare providers with easy-to-use office tools for patient education and charting documentation. Resources are provided within the text, with printable materials available on the enclosed CD-ROM for ready use in the clinic. Additional materials may be accessed through Dr. Marcus's website www.dawnmarcusmd.com. Both authors are eager to receive comments and suggestions for additions and improvements to the book through a link available at this website.

Pittsburgh, PA, USA   Dawn A. Marcus, MD
Madison, WI, USA   Philip A. Bain, MD

Contents

Chapter 1
Understanding Migraine and Pregnancy

Key Chapter Points

- One in five women experiences migraine during her reproductive years.
- Cycling estradiol levels predict migraine changes throughout a woman's reproductive years. Migraine is typically aggravated by low estradiol (e.g., premenstrual exacerbation) and improved with high estradiol (e.g., pregnancy).
- Migraine improves during pregnancy for about half of women. If improvement is going to occur, it usually does so before the end of the first trimester.
- Migraines typically reoccur after delivery, although breastfeeding may delay headache recurrence.

Keywords Breastfeeding · Lactation · Migraine · Nursing · Pregnancy · Trimester

> I've had bad migraines since I was a teenager and I just found out I'm pregnant. When I told my mother-in-law, she told me how much worse her headaches were when she was pregnant and that the doctor won't let you use any medications before the baby's born. I was so happy to finally be pregnant, but now I'm afraid I'll have nine miserable months in bed! HELP!

About half of all adults worldwide report having headaches [1]. Consequently, headache is one of the most common complaints seen in primary care. A survey of medical records from 289 randomly selected primary care patients in the United States found that nearly half of all patients reported a pain complaint [2]. The only somatic complaints more common than headache were back and lower extremity pain (Fig. 1.1). Furthermore, chart review one year later showed that the odds of having persistent somatic symptoms were twice as high among patients reporting headache or back pain.

Migraine is the most common benign, recurring headache seen in primary care offices and is distinguished from other common headaches by the occurrence of disabling symptoms (including pain, nausea, and sensitivity to lights and sounds) that persist for several hours or days (Table 1.1). An international panel reviewed records for 1,203 patients seeking treatment for headache in 128

D.A. Marcus, P.A. Bain, *Effective Migraine Treatment in Pregnant and Lactating Women: A Practical Guide*, DOI 10.1007/978-1-60327-439-5_1,
© Humana Press, a part of Springer Science+Business Media, LLC 2009

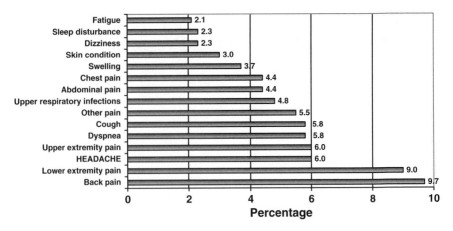

Fig. 1.1 Somatic complaints in primary care patients (Based on [2])
Somatic complaints endorsed by ≥2% of randomly-selected primary care patients are shown in the graph.

clinical practices [3]. Although migraine only affects about one in six people in the general population, among patients seeing their doctors for headache, 94% had migraine. Tension-type headache, though much more common than migraine, is rarely seen in the clinic as it is usually not disabling enough to warrant an office visit.

Table 1.1 Characteristics of common, recurring headaches

	Location	Typical duration (hours)	Usual behavior during headache
Migraine	Often but not always unilateral (affected side should vary at least occasionally). May become holocranial, especially when more severe	4–72	Reduced productivity, lies down, seeks dark and quiet isolation. May place washcloth over forehead and eyes and go to sleep. May be nauseated although vomiting usually only with very severe episodes.
Tension-type	Bilateral	8–24 or constant	No interference
Medication overuse	Bilateral	Constant with fluctuating severity	No interference
Cluster	Unilateral eye (always affecting the SAME side)	½–2	Agitated, avoids lying down, paces, smokes, showers, hits head

> **Pearl for the practitioner:**
> Migraine is the most common recurring headache seen in primary care. Tension-type headache, although more common than migraine, is rarely disabling enough to warrant a visit to the doctor.

Women are more than twice as likely to experience migraine as men, with migraine typically occurring between puberty and menopause. Because migraine predominates during the active reproductive years, questions about conception, pregnancy, and postnatal care are commonly addressed with women's healthcare providers. In general, regular changes in estrogen levels serve as an important migraine-activating trigger. Headaches often predictably worsen when estrogen levels drop from a high to a low level, such as with menstruation or after delivery (Fig. 1.2). Headaches will also often abate when estrogen levels are no longer changing from high to low levels, resulting in predictable improvements with pregnancy and menopause. Sustained elevations in estradiol, as with pregnancy, offer protection against headaches for many women. Furthermore, lack of cycling after menopause also tends to reduce migraine frequency and severity. Women often notice an unexpected worsening of migraine in the perimenopausal period when they are experiencing other somatic symptoms, like hot flashes. Headache aggravation at this time may be due to fluctuating estradiol levels. Migraine also tends to worsen after surgical menopause with hysterectomy/oophorectomy, while improving with spontaneous menopause [4]. Better outcome after natural menopause suggests a role for other factors in addition to lack of estrogen cycling. For example, reduced responsiveness of neural receptors to pain-provoking chemicals with aging seems to result in headache improvement in seniors for both men and women.

> **Pearl for the practitioner:**
> Fluctuating estrogen level is a potent headache trigger.

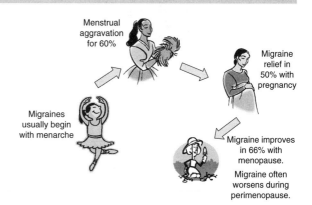

Fig. 1.2 Predicted migraine changes over a woman's reproductive lifetime

Migraine affects nearly one in five women in their reproductive years. Women with migraine are often concerned about how migraine will affect their pregnancies and whether they will be able to safely and effectively manage migraine episodes when pregnant and nursing. Fortunately, migraine improves in about half of women during pregnancy. Consequently, many doctors use a "wait-and-see" approach of delaying migraine treatment during pregnancy, in hopes of spontaneous improvement. While this viewpoint may seem prudent, failing to identify those patients who need more intensive treatment can result in unnecessary patient suffering, dehydration, disability, and overuse of over-the-counter medications.

> **Pearl for the practitioner:**
> Migraine improves for half of women during pregnancy. For those that do not, more intensive therapy is needed in order to avoid unnecessary patient suffering, dehydration, disability, and overuse of over-the-counter medications.

Although many women decide to restrict prescription migraine treatments during pregnancy, up to one in three pregnant women self-medicates for symptoms, especially with analgesics [5–7]. Healthcare providers must recognize the need to effectively treat symptoms, including troublesome headaches, during pregnancy. Fortunately, many effective treatment options are relatively safe to use when pregnant and breastfeeding. Available therapies include medication and non-medication treatments, traditional and alternative therapies, and nutritional supplements. By providing education and resources, as well as a consistent treatment strategy, pregnant women can be empowered to gain control over their headaches. Utilizing safer and effective therapies can improve the quality of the pregnancy experience and allow women to confidently breastfeed their infants while being treated for headaches.

> **Pearl for the practitioner:**
> Relatively safe and effective treatment options are available for the pregnant and lactating migraine sufferer.

This book describes expected changes in migraine patterns during pregnancy and breastfeeding. Treatments designed to reduce migraine pain during the attack and to prevent migraine attacks from occurring will be described, including medication, non-medication, complementary, and nutritional therapies. Headache diaries, patient educational tools, and detailed instructions for pain management and physical therapy exercises provided will help facilitate migraine treatment. This book will be a helpful resource for those who treat migraine sufferers who are pregnant and/or who choose to breastfeed their infants. Readers will develop a practical approach to the evaluation and treatment of the pregnant and lactating headache sufferer.

Typical Concerns Your Patient May Have

Your patient asks:

How do I know if I have migraines?

Migraines are disabling, intermittent headaches associated with sensitivity to environmental stimuli. A brief, non-physician-administered screening questionnaire (the Migraine Assessment Tool or MAT) is a validated tool for diagnosing migraine, with good reliability and stability with repeat administration (Fig. 1.3) [8]. This questionnaire can be effectively administered by healthcare personnel with no special expertise in the field of headache to identify patients with probable migraine.

> ***Pearl for the practitioner:***
> Migraine is a recurring, intermittent, disabling headache usually lasting 4–24 hours that is associated with nausea or light and sound sensitivity. Most headaches resulting in functional impairment are migraine.

Your patient asks:

What causes migraines?

Migraine is a common, controllable (not curable) biochemical condition of the brain, often referred to as a threshold disorder. When a genetically prone/susceptible patient is exposed to a headache trigger (whether identified or not), the threshold for the headache is exceeded and a cascade of events begins. Migraine sufferers experience an increased sensitivity to activation of pain-provoking pathways in the nervous system. Current theories about the physiology of migraine explain the occurrence of headache and other migraine features in response to activation of intracranial neural and vascular structures (Fig. 1.4). Exposure to internal and external triggers (including stress, changes in sleep and eating habits, and hormonal cycling) enhances intracranial activity of a variety of important headache-activating neurotransmitters, including nitric oxide, serotonin, and norepinephrine, which stimulate vascular dilation. Dilated intracranial, extracerebral blood vessels result in a perceived throbbing sensation and increased blood flow. More importantly, neurons surrounding these blood vessels become stretched, triggering the trigeminal system. Feedback signals, mediated by calcitonin gene-related peptide (CGRP), travel back along trigeminal fibers to intracranial, extracerebral

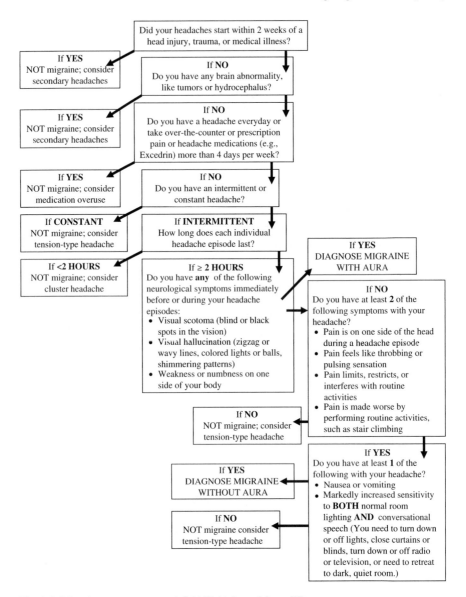

Fig. 1.3 Migraine-assessment tool (MAT) (Adapted from [8])

meningeal vessels, causing a positive feedback loop to perpetuate vascular dilation and trigeminal activation. The trigeminal system also activates the hypothalamus, possibly resulting in migraine-related cravings. Activation of cervical trigeminal structures may facilitate transmission to somatic neurons, resulting in muscle contraction. Signals also travel to the thalamus and cortex to relay pain messages.

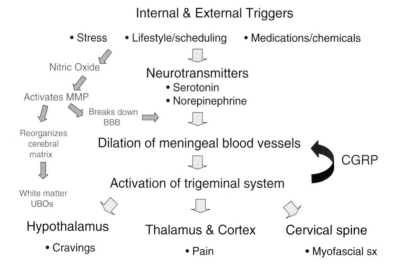

Fig. 1.4 Neurovascular model of migraine
CGRP = calcitonin gene-related peptide, MMP = matrix metalloprotease, sx = symptoms, UBO = unidentified bright objects.

Understanding changes in threshold that occur during migraine can help explain the usual time course of symptoms:

- Migraine begins with exposure to a trigger or activating factor that exceeds a migraine threshold and results in a cascade of complex events.
- Activation of the hypothalamus results in a feeling of general unease and cravings that often precede a migraine by several hours, called a prodrome.
- Auras of visual hallucinations may occur due to neural activation followed by cortical spreading depression in the occipital cortex.
- The painful stage of migraine occurs when meningeal blood vessels dilate, causing a throbbing sensation and activating trigeminal neurons to send pain messages. Trigeminal activation may also result in neck pain and excessive tenderness of the scalp and face, called cutaneous allodynia (skin-related pain from stimulation that would not normally be considered to be painful).
- Prolonged over-stimulation of neural structures may continue for several hours following pain resolution, resulting in a migraine postdrome of fatigue and feeling "hung over."

> ***Pearl for the practitioner:***
> Migraine is a threshold disorder. Numerous factors lower the threshold, making it easier for a headache to occur. Other factors, such as the migraine preventive medications, raise the threshold and make it harder for a headache to occur.

Nitric oxide also activates matrix metalloproteases (MMP), important compounds for brain development and plasticity. MMP-9 is linked to opening of the blood-brain barrier (BBB) and plays an important role in the pathogenesis of brain ischemia and possibly migraine. Cortical spreading depression at the onset of migraine results in upregulation of MMP-9 within 15–30 minutes that persists over 48 hours [9], causing breakdown of the BBB, edema, and vascular extravasation. These changes in brain fluid status may explain the occurrence of non-specific, unidentified bright objects in the white matter on magnetic resonance imaging studies in about 30% of migraineurs. These effects may also help explain how medications and neurotransmitters outside of the BBB can gain access to the brain during a migraine.

Sex hormones, like estrogen, play a critical role in headache susceptibility by acting as an important neurotransmitter regulator. Vulnerability to a headache episode depends on a balance between headache-protecting neurotransmitters (serotonin, gamma amino-butyric acid [GABA], and endorphins) and headache-provoking neurochemicals (dopamine and norepinephrine). When concentration and activity of headache protectors outweigh that for headache producers, the patient is less susceptible to headache episodes (Fig. 1.5).

A. Neurovascular balancing act

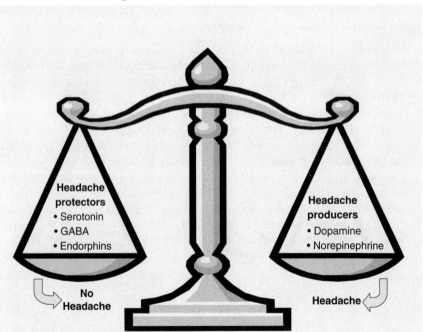

Fig. 1.5 Estrogen's effect on headache susceptibility
Solid lines represent increased or enhanced neurotransmitter activity, while dashed lines signify decreased or dampened neurotransmitter activity.

B. Stress modulates headache chemicals

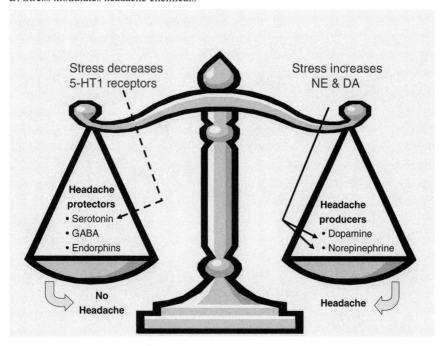

C. Treatment modulates headache chemicals

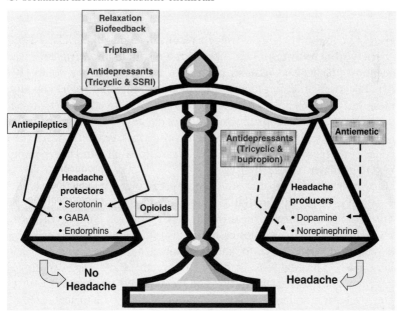

Fig. 1.5 (continued)

D. Estrogen modulates headache chemicals

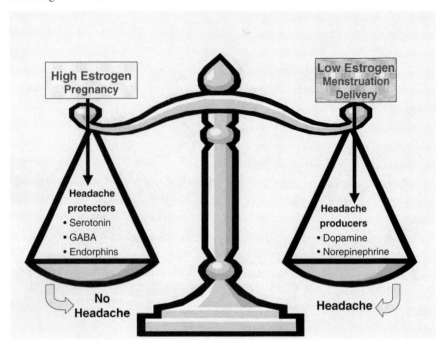

Fig. 1.5 (continued)

Exposure to common headache triggers results in changes in levels and activity of a variety of neurotransmitters. Stress, the most common trigger, increases headache producers and reduces protective activity from serotonin [10–12]. Both medication and non-medication migraine therapies work by directly affecting this neurochemical balance. Estrogen also directly affects levels and activity of both headache-producing and headache-protecting neurotransmitters. Elevated estrogen increases headache protectors, reducing headache risk. Conversely, decreases in estrogen levels increase dopamine and norepinephrine, increasing headache susceptibility.

Estrogen levels rise throughout human pregnancy, dropping precipitously after delivery. A longitudinal study monitored hormone levels in 52 primigravida women on normal diets during each trimester and 1 year postpartum. Compared to first trimester levels, estradiol increased six-fold by the third trimester, returning to almost undetectable levels after delivery (Fig. 1.6) [13]. The relationship between pain threshold and estradiol levels during pregnancy was evaluated in gonadectomized rats treated with estradiol in levels to simulate the typical rat pregnancy or a placebo (Fig. 1.7) [14]. The pain threshold in hormone-supplemented rats increased in concert with increasing estradiol levels, reaching a maximum with peak estradiol

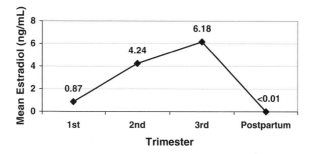

Fig. 1.6 Changes in estradiol levels during pregnancy and after delivery (Based on [13])
Pregnancy estradiol levels were measured at gestational weeks 12 (1st trimester), 22 (2nd trimester), and 32 (third trimester), with gestational dates confirmed by ultrasound. Postpartum estradiol was obtained 1 year after delivery.

levels at the time of the theoretical birth and rapidly reverting to baseline as estradiol levels fell after the theoretical birth. These same changes may also be identified during human pregnancy. The increased pain threshold noted in the second and third trimesters (related to high levels of estradiol) is the primary reason why headaches are far less common during this portion of pregnancy. As estrogen levels fall postpartum, the pain threshold also drops, resulting in return of headache episodes.

Breastfeeding may influence migraine by increasing levels of oxytocin and vasopressin [15], both of which increase the pain threshold. In rodent

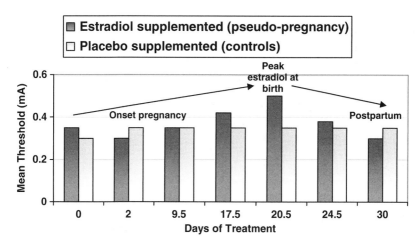

Fig. 1.7 Relationship between pain threshold and estradiol during simulated rat pregnancy (Based on [14])
Pregnancy was simulated by daily injections with estradiol to match levels typically achieved during a rodent pregnancy, or with a placebo. Mean threshold was measured repeatedly in both rodent groups.

experiments, central administration of either oxytocin or vasopressin increases the pain threshold, with this effect mediated by endogenous opioids [16–18]. Similar effects may occur in humans and explain the pain-protective effect of nursing. For example, a pilot study demonstrated both reduction in acute pain in 87% and headache prevention in 41% of migraineurs treated with vasopressin [19]. Consequently, breastfeeding might be expected to result in decreased pain sensitivity.

> ***Pearl for the practitioner:***
> Migraine is caused by an imbalance in brain neurochemicals like serotonin, gamma amino-butyric acid, dopamine, and norepinephrine. This imbalance is accentuated by fluctuating estrogen levels. Rising estrogen in later pregnancy offers a headache protective effect; while dropping estrogen levels with delivery precipitates headaches.

Your patient asks:

Why are women affected by migraines?

Estrogen is the primary female hormone that is responsible for a girl's development into a woman. When estrogen begins to cycle after puberty, changes in this hormone also help modify pain perception. Once estradiol levels begin to cycle, significant drops in estradiol can act as a reliable migraine trigger in many women, such as with menses and following delivery [20]. Monthly changes in estradiol and corresponding temporary reductions in pain thresholds during menses may explain why women have more aches and pains, like back pain, joint aches, and headaches, with their periods. Estrogen levels skyrocket during the end of pregnancy in preparation for childbirth, effectively elevating the pain threshold associated with both delivery pain and other pains, like migraine.

About two of every three women with migraine notice a strong link between their migraines and their reproductive cycle, noticing that their migraines:

- Began with menarche;
- Worsen with monthly periods;
- Improve in the second half of pregnancy;
- Worsen after delivery;
- Worsen during the perimenopause when other somatic symptoms, like hot flashes, are occurring;
- Improve during later menopause.

Women who have experienced menstrual changes with their migraines are more likely to report reduced migraine during pregnancy. Prior to conception, patients should track their migraines and menstrual periods for at least 3 cycles to determine whether there is a menstrual link for their headaches.

Hormonally-triggered migraines should occur when estradiol levels are dropping, typically on those 5 perimenstrual days associated with declining estradiol (2 days before until 2 days after the onset of menstrual flow). This pattern should occur in at least 2 of 3 consecutive menstrual cycles. Fig. 1.8A shows a

A. Sample diary

Day	Migraine Severity				Menstrual Day
	None	Mild	Moderate	Severe	
Sunday					
Morning					
Noon					
Evening					
Bedtime					
Monday					
Morning					
Noon					
Evening					
Bedtime					
Tuesday					
Morning					
Noon					
Evening					
Bedtime					
Wednesday					
Morning					
Noon					
Evening					
Bedtime					

Fig. 1.8 Diary to determine menstrual link to migraines

Thursday					
Morning					
Noon					
Evening					
Bedtime					
Friday					
Morning					
Noon					
Evening					
Bedtime					
Saturday					
Morning					
Noon					
Evening					
Bedtime					

Record migraine severity 4 times daily . Record if you are experiencing your menstrual period on each day once daily.

Fig. 1.8 (continued)

B. Completed diary suggesting menstrual relationship

Day	Migraine Severity				Menstrual Day
	None	Mild	Moderate	Severe	
Sunday					no
Morning	X				
Noon	X				
Evening	X				
Bedtime	X				
Monday					no
Morning	X				
Noon	X				
Evening	X				
Bedtime	X				
Tuesday					yes
Morning	X				
Noon	X				
Evening	X				
Bedtime		X			
Wednesday					yes
Morning				X	
Noon				X	
Evening				X	
Bedtime			X		

Fig. 1.8 (continued)

Thursday						yes
Morning		X				
Noon		X				
Evening		X				
Bedtime	X					
Friday						yes
Morning	X					
Noon	X					
Evening	X					
Bedtime	X					
Saturday						yes
Morning	X					
Noon	X					
Evening	X					
Bedtime	X					

This patient consistently recorded migraines occurring during the first 2 days after beginning her period, suggesting a relationship to hormonal changes.

Fig. 1.8 (continued)

C. Completed diary suggesting no menstrual relationship

Day	Migraine Severity				Menstrual Day
	None	Mild	Moderate	Severe	
Sunday					no
Morning	X				
Noon	X				
Evening		X			
Bedtime				X	
Monday					
Morning	X				
Noon	X				
Evening	X				
Bedtime	X				
Tuesday					no
Morning				X	
Noon				X	
Evening			X		
Bedtime	X				
Wednesday					no
Morning	X				
Noon	X				
Evening	X				
Bedtime	X				

Fig. 1.8 (continued)

Thursday						no
Morning	X					
Noon	X					
Evening	X					
Bedtime	X					
Friday						yes
Morning	X					
Noon	X					
Evening	X					
Bedtime	X					
Saturday						yes
Morning			X			
Noon				X		
Evening				X		
Bedtime	X					

Migraines occurred about 2-3 days each week in this patient, with no increase in likelihood of occurrence or severity during the early perimenstrual days when estradiol levels drop to levels that may provoke migraine. Her migraines are not linked to hormonal changes.

Fig. 1.8 (continued)

sample diary to record headache and menstrual activity. Fig. 1.8B shows migraine aggravation occurring in relation to menses, while the patient recording the diary in Fig. 1.8C shows migraine occurring coincidentally with menses. In this latter patient, migraine occurred randomly throughout the menstrual cycle, with no predilection for early menstrual days when estradiol levels are low and most likely to act as a migraine trigger.

> *Pearl for the practitioner:*
> Women who have experienced menstrual changes with their migraines are more likely to report reduced migraine during pregnancy.

Your patient asks:

I have migraines and my husband and I would like to become pregnant within the next year. What should I do to get ready for this?

Planning for pregnancy in a patient with migraine is important. Headache control should be maximized prior to conception, continuing adequate contraception while developing a program to minimize frequency and severity of headaches. When the headache pattern is stable, medications can be switched to those that are safer in pregnancy and contraception can be stopped. In addition, effective non-drug approaches (e.g., biofeedback, stress reduction strategies, trigger identification and avoidance, etc.) can and should be learned and mastered in the preconception phase to permit minimizing medication needs during conception and pregnancy. Furthermore, all women capable of becoming pregnant should take a multivitamin with an adequate amount of folate (at least 400 micrograms daily) to prevent neural tube defects. Once contraception is no longer being used, the migraineur should be treated as if she were pregnant, utilizing medications known to be relatively safe in pregnancy, such as metoclopramide and ondansetron for nausea and acetaminophen for pain. Regular follow-ups should occur once pregnancy has been confirmed.

Your patient asks:

Will my migraines get worse when I'm pregnant?

Primary headaches, especially migraine, typically improve during the first trimester of pregnancy, when estrogen levels are rising most dramatically. Retrospective studies report spontaneous improvement in 50–80% of pregnant women with migraine and 30% with tension-type headache [21–24]. A recent prospective study collected headache information on 1,101 women during their pregnancies [25]. Either pre-existing or current headache was reported for 97% of women, with pre-existing headaches usually migraine (85%) or tension-type headache (11%). Only 7% of women reported developing their first headache or a new headache with the current pregnancy. About one in three women with her first or a new headache during this pregnancy was diagnosed with migraine and one in three was diagnosed with headache attributed to hypertension. The only other diagnoses occurring in >5% of patients were non-specific headache (7%), cervicogenic headache (6%), and rhinosinusitis (5%). As predicted by retrospective studies, most women experienced headache improvement over the course of pregnancy, with two-thirds of women reporting improvement during their third trimester (Fig. 1.9).

Although most women do experience headache improvement with pregnancy, women reporting ongoing headaches at the end of the first trimester (usually the first obstetrical visit) are unlikely to experience significant headache improvement during the remainder of pregnancy. A small prospective study of 30 mixed headache sufferers experiencing recurring primary headache at the end of the first trimester showed only an additional 30% improvement between

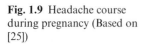

Fig. 1.9 Headache course during pregnancy (Based on [25])

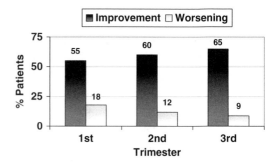

the 2nd and 3rd trimesters, with a slightly greater likelihood of improvement in women with migraine [26]. These data suggest that more intensive treatment should be offered to women with headaches persisting into the second trimester rather than monitoring for spontaneous improvement.

Even when primary headaches improve with pregnancy, they typically recur soon after delivery. In a prospective study of 49 pregnant women with a migraine diagnosis, migraine occurred within two days of delivery for 4% of women, within one week for 34%, and within one month for 55% [27]. Breast-feeding decreased risk for headache recurrence within both the first week and first month postpartum.

> **Pearl for the practitioner:**
> Women reporting headaches at the end of the first trimester (usually the first obstetrical visit) are unlikely to experience significant headache improvement during the remainder of pregnancy and should be offered treatment.

Your patient asks:

How do I know that my pregnancy headaches aren't caused by a serious illness?

Headaches during pregnancy are usually caused by benign, primary headaches (especially migraine and tension-type). In some cases, however, headaches may be caused by other medical conditions (Table 1.2). Secondary causes of headache during pregnancy include infections, eclampsia/preeclampsia, vascular disease (e.g., aneurysms, dissections, and arteriovenous malformations), and increased intracranial pressure. Acute strokes, cerebral venous thrombosis, symptomatic brain tumor, and benign intracranial hypertension (pseudotumor cerebri) occur with increased frequency during pregnancy [28]. Pregnancy is also associated with increased risk of subarachnoid hemorrhage, typically from ruptured arteriovenous malformations and postpartum cerebral venous thrombosis [28]. Cerebral venous thrombosis occurs in 10–20 women/100,000 deliveries [29,30]. Nearly 80% of cases occur during the first two postpartum weeks, with 8%

Table 1.2 Headaches influenced by pregnancy

Benign	Pathologic
Migraine	Preeclapmsia and eclampsia
Tension-type	Stroke (hemorrhagic and thrombotic)
Analgesic overuse	Arteriovenous malformations
	Brain tumors (e.g., pituitary adenomas and meningiomas)
	Benign intracranial hypertension

occurring during the third trimester and another 8% after two postpartum weeks [31]. While tumor incidence does not increase with pregnancy, the growth of pituitary adenomas and meningiomas is accelerated during pregnancy [32,33]. Benign intracranial hypertension (pseudotumor cerebri) may also be triggered by elevated estrogen, and may occur or worsen during pregnancy [34–36].

New headaches or significant change in headache activity during pregnancy requires a detailed history and physical examination to differentiate benign, primary headaches from pathological headaches. Headache associated with papilledema, focal neurological signs or symptoms, or seizures suggests intracranial pathology and necessitates a complete neurological evaluation. Conditions that may mimic migraine during pregnancy and postpartum include: low pressure headache related to spinal anesthesia, eclampsia/preeclampsia, cerebral venous thrombosis, subarachnoid hemorrhage, intracranial tumors, idiopathic intracranial hypertension (pseudotumor cerebri), and meningitis.

In a retrospective review of 63 pregnant women reporting to an emergency department for a primary complaint of headache, magnetic resonance or computed tomography studies were normal or revealed only incidental/non-specific findings in most of these women (73%) [37]. Pathological conditions included sinusitis (8%), cerebral venous thrombosis (6%), reversible posterior leukoencephalopathy/eclampsia (6%), pseudotumor (3%), and intracranial hemorrhage (3%). Among patients with abnormal neurological examinations, a pathological condition was identified in 38% of patients. Among patients with normal neurological examinations, a pathological scan occurred in 19% of patients. Therefore, although the presence of an abnormal neurological exam predicts increased likelihood of intracranial pathology, absence of an abnormal examination alone does not provide adequate assurance of no intracranial pathology. Recommendations for safely evaluating new or worrisome headaches during pregnancy are provided in Chapter 9.

> ***Pearl for the practitioner:***
> Most headaches encountered in pregnant patients are benign. Secondary headaches such as those caused by infections, preeclampsia/eclampsia, vascular disease, and increased intracranial pressure are much less common, but should be kept in mind when assessing a pregnant woman with headaches.

Your patient asks:

Will having migraines complicate my pregnancy?

Migraineurs are at increased risk for developing pregnancy-related hypertension. In a case-controlled study, the occurrence of primary headache was compared in 75 women experiencing pregnancy-induced hypertension with proteinuria (preeclampsia) and 75 women with uncomplicated pregnancies, matched for age and parity [38]. A history of migraine was endorsed by 59% with eclampsia and 17% without, with tension-type headache in 4% with eclampsia and 7% without. These data suggest a link between migraine and preeclampsia.

Migraine, especially migraine with aura, has also been linked to an increased risk for developing ischemic stroke [39]. Pregnancy is similarly associated with increased occurrence of thrombotic events, such as stroke. Using data from the Nationwide Inpatient Sample for the Healthcare Cost and Utilization Project of the Agency for Healthcare Research and Quality, stroke was identified at a rate of 34.2 per 100,000 deliveries [40]. In this survey, migraine was a strong independent risk factor for pregnancy-related stroke (odds ratio = 16.9). Other strong predictor factors included diagnoses of systemic lupus erythematosus (odds ratio = 15.2) and thrombophilia (odds ratio = 16.0).

> **Pearl for the practitioner:**
> Migraine sufferers are at increased risk for developing preeclampsia/eclampsia and ischemic stroke, though these events are still quite uncommon.

Your patient asks:

Will it hurt the baby if I have a migraine when I'm pregnant?

Fortunately, babies born to women with migraine have no apparent increased risk for developing congenital malformations [41,42]. A recent report compared outcome in 38,151 newborns, 713 of whom had been born to mothers with severe migraine during pregnancy [43]. Mean gestational age and birth weight, as well as the percentage of babies with preterm delivery or low birth weight, were similar between infants born to mothers with and without severe migraine during pregnancy.

Suboptimal maternal nutrition in early pregnancy may affect fetal growth and development [44]. Although most studies evaluating the effects of nutritional deficits or dehydration during pregnancy are related to nausea and vomiting from hyperemesis gravidarum, severe and frequent migraine may also contribute to dehydration and periods of poor nutrition. Preventing dehydration and ensuring good nutrition are important factors for deciding to use headache medications during pregnancy.

Pearl for the practitioner:
Babies born to women with migraine have no identified increased risk for
congenital malformations.

Your patient asks:

Can I still breastfeed if I have migraines?

Breastfeeding can result in decreased headache frequency and severity. This, as
well as the multiple known health benefits of breastfeeding, should be emphasized
to the woman considering breastfeeding her infant. A large series of over 2,500
migraineurs showed that headaches are very rarely worsened with lactation [45].

Pearl for the practitioner:
Migraine recurrence after delivery is typically delayed in women who
breastfeed compared with non-breastfeeding women.

Your patient asks:

Will I be able to use my migraine medication when I'm pregnant or nursing?

Many migraine medications are available and relatively safe for use during
pregnancy and breastfeeding. Chapters 4, 5, 6, and 7 in this book describe in
detail migraine treatments that offer effective headache control during pregnancy
and lactation. Clinicians should remember, however, that the term *safe* denotes
relative safety, based on sometimes limited available data in women during
pregnancy and breastfeeding. All medications are associated with some adverse
events. Ideally, the clinician chooses those therapies that minimize safety concerns while maximizing efficacy. Patients should understand that all medications
used during pregnancy or when nursing should be taken judiciously with healthcare provider supervision to ensure the safest possible therapy.

Pearl for the practitioner:
While headache medications are restricted during pregnancy and while
nursing, there are a number of safer and effective options.

Your patient asks:

How can I tell if my migraines are getting worse during my pregnancy?

Patients can monitor their response to therapy by using headache calendars or
diaries (sample provided in Chapter 10). Recording headache frequency and
severity helps to assess patterns that can aid in treatment planning. Logging
headache severity several times daily helps provide important information

about headache duration that will be missed if patients only record severity once daily. Diaries are especially important during pregnancy to ensure and document that the benefits from treatment outweigh any possible negative effects from treatment.

Your patient asks:

I heard migraines are genetic. Am I going to pass along my migraines to my baby?

Headaches, including migraine, tend to run in families. In a recent sample of 5,474 German households, parental headache was strongly linked to pediatric headache [46]. In this sample, when a biological parent experienced headaches, 72% of the children also reported headaches. Conversely, if neither parent had headaches, only 28% of children had headaches.

A family history of headache is particularly strong among migraineurs. Several candidate genes have been identified as possible sites of a migraine locus (Box 1.1) [47–50]. One in three people with migraine will have at least one first-degree relative (parent, sibling, or child) who also has migraine [51]. In general, if only one parent gets migraines, there is a 50% chance his or her children will also develop migraine [52]. When both parents suffer from migraines, their child has a 75% percent chance of also becoming a migraineur.

Pearl for the practitioner:
When one parent has migraine, the child has a 50% chance of developing migraine. When both parents have migraines, the child's risk increases to 75%.

Box 1.1 Identified chromosomal linkages for migraine

- Familial hemiplegic migraine
- 19p13
  - Brain-specific P/Q-type calcium channel α1-subunit (CACNA1A)
- 1q31 and 1q23
  - α2 subunit of Na^+/K^+ pump (ATP1A2)
- 2q24
  - Neuronal voltage-gated Na^+ channel (SCN1A)
- Migraine with aura
- 4q24
- 19p13
  - Not CACNA1A region
- Migraine without aura
- 14q21.2-q22.3

Summary

Migraine affects one in five women during their reproductive years. Cycling estradiol levels affect the threshold for migraine, with headache susceptibility increased when estradiol levels drop to low levels (e.g., premenstrual exacerbation) and decreased when estradiol levels are elevated (e.g., pregnancy). Consequently, migraine improves during pregnancy for about half of women. If improvement is going to occur, it usually does so before the end of the first trimester. Migraines typically reoccur after delivery, although breastfeeding may delay headache recurrence. Prior to becoming pregnant, fertile women should be counseled about safer treatments to use during conception and pregnancy. Safer and effective medication and non-medication treatment options are available to help control headaches during conception, pregnancy, and lactation.

Practical pointers

- Migraine is the most common headache seen in primary care, including during pregnancy and lactation. Tension-type headaches are more common in the general population, but rarely result in a visit to the doctor.
- History and examination can readily rule out important causes of secondary headache.
- Migraine improves for half of women during pregnancy, with improvement usually occurring during the first trimester.
- Babies born to women with migraine have no increased risk for congenital malformations.
- Preconception counseling should include maximizing headache control while contraception is still being used, then converting to therapies that are safer to use during conception and pregnancy before discontinuing contraception.
- While headache medications are restricted during pregnancy and nursing, there are a number of relatively safe and effective options.
- Migraines typically recur after delivery, although nursing delays return of headaches for many women.
- Migraines are often inherited. If mom or dad suffers from migraines, the baby has a 50% chance of later developing migraine. If both parents have migraines, the baby's risk increases to 75%.

References

1. Stovner LJ, Hagen K, Jensen R, et al. The global burden of headache: a documentation of headache prevalence and disability worldwide. *Cephalalgia* 2007;27: 193–210.
2. Khan AA, Khan A, Harezlak J, Tu W, Kroenke K. Somatic symptoms in primary care: etiology and outcome. *Psychosomatics* 2003;44:471–478.

3. Tepper SJ, Dahlöf CH, Dowson A, et al. Prevalence and diagnosis of migraine in patients consulting their physician with a complaint of headache: data from the Landmark study. *Headache* 2004;44:856–864.
4. Neri I, Granella F, Nappi R, Manzoni GC, Facchinetti F, Genazzani AR. Characteristics of headache at menopause: a clinico-epidemiologic study. *Maturitas* 1993;17:31–37.
5. Gomes KR, Moron AF, Silva R, Siqueira AA. Prevalence of use of medicines during pregnancy and its relationship to maternal factors. *Rev Saude Publica* 1999;33:246–254.
6. Damase-Michel C, Lapeyre-Mestre M, Moly C, Fournie A, Montastruc JL. Drug use during pregnancy: survey in 250 women consulting at a university hospital center. *J Gynecol Obstet Biol Repro (Paris)* 2000;29:77–85.
7. Fonseca MR, Fonseca E, Bergsten-Mendes G. Prevalence of drug use during pregnancy: a pharmacoepidemiological approach. *Rev Saude Publica* 2002;36:205–212.
8. Marcus DA, Kapelewski C, Jacob RG, Rudy TE, Furman JM. Validation of a brief nurse-administered migraine assessment tool. *Headache* 2004;44:328–332.
9. Gursoy-Ozdemir Y. Cortical spreading depression activates and upregulates MMP-9. *J Clin Investigation* 2004;113:1447–1455.
10. Haleem DJ, Saify ZS, Siddiqui S, Batool F, Haleem MA. Pre- and post-synaptic responses to 1-(1-naphthylpiperazine) following adaptation to stress in rats. *Prog Neuropsycho Biol Psychiatry* 2002;26:149–156.
11. von Kanel R, Mills PJ, Ziegler MG, Dimsdale JE. Effect of beta2-adrenergic receptor functioning and increased norepinephrine on the hypercoaguable state with mental stress. *Am Heart J* 2002;144:68–72.
12. Moghaddam B. Stress activation of glutamate neurotransmission in the prefrontal cortex: implications for dopamine-associated psychiatric disorders. *Biol Psychiatry* 2002;51:775–787.
13. Soldin OP, Guo T, Weiderpass E, et al. Steroid hormone levels in pregnancy and 1 year postpartum using isotope dilution tandem mass spectrometry. *Fertil Steril* 2005;84:701–710.
14. Dawson-Basoa MB, Gintzler AR. 17-Beta-estradiol and progesterone modulate an intrinsic opioid analgesic system. *Brain Res* 1993;601:241–245.
15. Fischer D, Latchev VK, Hellback S, Hassan AS, Almeida OX. Lactation as a model of naturally reversible hypercorticalism plasticity in the mechanisms governing hypothalamo-pituitary-adrenocortical activity in rats. *J Clin Invest* 1995;96:1208–1215.
16. Yang J. Intrathecal administration of oxytocin induces analgesia in low back pain involving the endogenous opiate peptide system. *Spine* 1994;19:867–871.
17. Yang J, Yang Y, Chen J, et al. Central oxytocin enhances antinociception in the rat. *Peptides* 2007;28:1113–1119.
18. Yang J, Yang Y, Xu HT, et al. Arginine vasopressin induces periaqueductal gray release of enkephalin and endorphin relating to pain modulation in the rat. *Regul Pept* 2007;142:29–36.
19. Lobzin VS, Vasil'ev NS. Lechenie migreni vazopressinom. *Zh Nevropatol Psikhiatr* 1989;1:54–58.
20. Lichten EM, Lichten JB, Whitty A, Pieper D. The confirmation of a biochemical marker for women's hormonal migraine: the depo-estradiol challenge test. *Headache* 1996;36:367–371.
21. Callaghan N. The migraine syndrome in pregnancy. *Neurology* 1968;18:197–199.
22. Granella F, Sances G, Zanferrari C, et al. Migraine without aura and reproductive life events: a clinical epidemiological study in 1300 women. *Headache* 1993;33:385–389.
23. Chen TC, Leviton A. Headache recurrences in pregnant women with migraine. *Headache* 1994;34:107–110.
24. Maggiono F, Alessi C, Maggino T, et al. Primary headaches and pregnancy. *Cephalalgia* 1995;15:54.

25. Melhado EM, Maciel JA, Guerreiro CM. Headache during gestation: evaluation of 1101 women. *Can J Neurol Sci* 2007;34:187–192.
26. Marcus DA, Scharff L, Turk DC. Longitudinal prospective study of headache during pregnancy and postpartum. *Headache* 1999;39:625–632.
27. Sances G, Granella F, Nappi RE, et al. Course of migraine during pregnancy and postpartum: a prospective study. *Cephalalgia* 2003;23:197–205.
28. Marcus DA. Headache in pregnancy. *Curr Pain Headache Rep* 2003;7:288–296.
29. Francois P, Fabre M, Lioret E, Jan M. Vascular cerebral thrombosis during pregnancy and post-partum. *Neurochirurgie* 2000;46:105–109.
30. Lanska DJ, Kryscio RJ. Stroke and intracranial venous thrombosis during pregnancy and puerperium. *Neurology* 1998;51:1622–1628.
31. Panagariya A, Maru A. Cerebral venous thrombosis in pregnancy and puerperium – a prospective study. *J Assoc Physicians India* 1997;45:857–859.
32. Azpilcueta A, Peral C, Giraldo I, Chen FJ, Contreras G. Meningioma in pregnancy. Report of a case and review of the literature. *Ginecol Obstet Mex* 1995;63:349–351.
33. Saitoh Y, Oku Y, Izumoto S, Go J. Rapid growth of a meningioma during pregnancy: relationship with estrogen and progesterone receptors – case report. *Neurol Med Cir (Tokyo)* 1989;29:440–443.
34. Arseni C, Simoca I, Jipescu I, Leventi E, Grecu P, Sima A. Pseudotumor cerebri: risk factors, clinical course, prognostic criteria. *Rom J Neurol Psychiatry* 1992;30:115–132.
35. Katz VL, Peterson R, Cefalo RC. Pseudotumor cerebri and pregnancy. *Am J Perinatol* 1989;6:442–445.
36. Koontz WL, Herbert WP, Cefalo RC. Pseudotumor cerebri in pregnancy. *Obstet Gynecol* 1983;62:324–327.
37. Ramchandren S, Cross BJ, Liebeskind DS. Emergent headaches during pregnancy: correlation between neurologic examination and neuroimaging. *Am J Neuroradiol* 2007;28:1085–1087.
38. Facchinetti F, Allais G, D'Amico R, Benedetto C, Volpe A. The relationship between headache and preeclampsia: a case-control study. *Eur J Obstet Gynecol Repro Bio* 2005;121:143–148.
39. Kurth T. Associations between migraine and cardiovascular disease. *Expert Rev Neurother* 2007;7:1097–1104.
40. James AH, Bushnell CD, Jamison MG, Myers ER. Incidence and risk factors for stroke in pregnancy and the puerperium. *Obstet Gynecol* 2005;106:509–516.
41. Wainscott G, Sullivan FM, Volans GN, Wilkinson M. The outcome of pregnancy in women suffering from migraine. *Postgrad Med J* 1978;54:98–102.
42. O'Quinn S, Ephross SA, Williams V, et al. Pregnancy and perinatal outcomes in migraineurs using sumatriptan: a prospective study. *Arch Gynecol Obstet* 1999;263:7–12.
43. Bànhidy F, Acs N, Horváth-Puhó E, Czeizel AE. Pregnancy complications and delivery outcomes in pregnant women with severe migraine. *Eur J Obstet Gynecol Reprod Biol* 2007;134:157–163.
44. Coad J, Al-Rasasi B, Morgan J. Nutrient insult in early pregnancy. *Proc Nutr Soc* 2002;61:51–59.
45. Wall VR. Breastfeeding and migraine headaches. *J Hum Lact* 1992;8:209–212.
46. Kröner-Herwig B, Heinrich M, Morris L. Headache in German children and adolescents: a population-based epidemiological study. *Cephalalgia* 2007;27:519–527.
47. Hershey AD. Genetics of migraine headache in children. *Curr Pain Headache Rep* 2007;11:390–395.
48. Wessman M, Kallela M, Kaunisto MA, et al. A susceptibilty locus for migraine with aura, on chromosome 4q24. *Am J Hum Genet* 2002;70:652–662.

49. Soragna D, Vettori A, Carraro G, et al. A locus for migraine without aura maps on chromosome 14q21.2-q22.3, *Am J Hum Genet* 2003;72:161–167.
50. Jones KW, Ehm MG, Pericak-Vance MA, et al. Migraine with aura susceptibility locus on chromosome 19p13 is distinct from the familial hemiplegic migraine locus. *Genomics* 2001;78:150–154.
51. Stewart WF, Bigal ME, Kolodner K, et al. Familial risk of migraine. Variation by proband age at onset and headache severity. *Neurology* 2006;66:344–348.
52. Eidelman D. What is the genetic factor in migraine? *Med Hypotheses* 2002;59:316–320.

Chapter 2
Safety Rating Systems for Drugs Used in Pregnancy and Lactation

Key Chapter Points

- The most widely used systems for categorizing drug risk during pregnancy in the United States are the Food and Drug Administration (FDA) and Teratogen Information System (TERIS) pregnancy risk classifications.
- Controlled data on using medications during pregnancy and lactation are lacking, making firm recommendations more difficult.
- Only fair agreement on risk category assignment exists when comparing common pregnancy risk classification systems within and between countries.
- Pregnancy risk categories should be used as general guidelines to help choose safer medication alternatives.
- Useful print and Internet resources help guide rational medication selections during pregnancy and lactation.

Keywords FDA · Risk · Teratogen · TERIS

This first-time mom excitedly told her family doctor that she had decided to "get super healthy" during her pregnancy, exercising regularly, eating only organic foods, and avoiding most medications. "I read that the FDA says drugs are safe during pregnancy when they're drug category A. So what can you prescribe for me that will control my migraines and be safe for the baby?"

Use of medications in pregnant and lactating women can be challenging for the clinician, who must carefully balance effectively treating migraines with limiting exposure to maternal medications by the fetus or breastfeeding infant. Making recommendations is compromised by the paucity of controlled studies directly testing drugs in pregnant and nursing women. Most available safety information is gleaned from animal studies, retrospective analyses, case reports, and epidemiological data, all of which have significant limitations.

Statistics about human pregnancy-related risks with prescription and nonprescription medications are most commonly derived from epidemiological study data obtained through cohort or case-controlled studies. Cohort studies compare adverse pregnancy outcomes between large groups of women exposed

D.A. Marcus, P.A. Bain, *Effective Migraine Treatment in Pregnant and Lactating Women: A Practical Guide*, DOI 10.1007/978-1-60327-439-5_2, © Humana Press, a part of Springer Science+Business Media, LLC 2009

to a potential toxin and women not exposed. Case-controlled studies evaluate maternal factors in children with and without a specific developmental abnormality. Cohort studies generally provide a more representative population sample, although large sample sizes are usually needed to identify an increased frequency of negative pregnancy outcomes. Post-marketing data obtained through pregnancy registries can also provide valuable information about pregnancy-related drug effects, although participation in these registries is voluntary, thus limiting data interpretation. Data are currently available for several migraine therapies using large, European epidemiological surveys and pharmaceutical company-sponsored exposure registries.

Despite the lack of ideal drug toxicology data during pregnancy and lactation, careful interpretation of available animal and human studies has resulted in the development of several widely accepted risk rating systems designed to facilitate safe drug recommendations during pregnancy and while nursing. This chapter will provide information on drug risk determination during pregnancy and nursing, explain commonly used risk classification systems and their shortcomings, and provide resources to assist the clinician when making important decisions about medication selection.

> **Pearl for the practitioner:**
> While controlled trials directly testing medications during pregnancy and lactation are lacking, useful resources and rating systems are available to help guide the clinician to make prudent choices when selecting medications.

Pregnancy

Medication Use During Pregnancy

Although women usually tell their doctors that they want to avoid medication during pregnancy, the vast majority of pregnant women consume both prescription and non-prescription medications. In one survey, 578 obstetric patients were interviewed about their medication use [1]. Prescription medications (excluding vitamin, mineral, and iron supplements) were used by 60% of women, over-the-counter medications by 93%, and herbal remedies by 45% (Fig. 2.1). The four most commonly prescribed categories of medications were: antibiotics (used by 35% of patients), respiratory drugs (15%), gastrointestinal products (13%), and opioids (8%). The most commonly used over-the-counter drugs were analgesics: acetaminophen (76%), ibuprofen (15%), and aspirin (2%). Herbal remedies were usually peppermint for nausea (18%) and cranberry for urinary tract symptoms (13%). Clinicians may be unaware that their patients are using over-the-counter therapies or prescriptions from

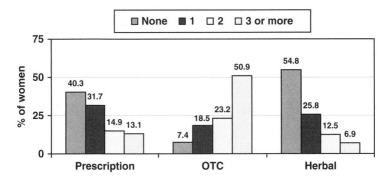

Fig. 2.1 Number of drugs used by pregnant women (Based on [1])
Prescription medications category excludes vitamin, folate, and iron supplementation.
OTC = over-the-counter medications.

other providers; consequently, healthcare providers must directly and explicitly ask patients about all prescription and non-prescription medications they are using.

> *Pearl for the practitioner:*
> Prescription medications (excluding vitamin, mineral, and iron supplements) are used by nearly two in every three women during pregnancy. Herbal remedies are used by nearly half, and almost all women will use over-the-counter medications when pregnant. Clinicians must directly ask patients about the use of both prescription and non-prescription treatments.

Epidemiological studies further disclose that a substantial minority of pregnant women use potentially harmful medications. Prescription records were reviewed for over 200,000 women in the Netherlands from 1995 to 2001 [2]. Among the 7,500 pregnant women included in this analysis, prescription medications were used by 86% of women when considering all prescriptions and 69% if vitamins, folate, and iron were excluded. Although most medications prescribed to pregnant women were considered safe, 21% of pregnant women were prescribed potentially harmful medications and 9% received prescriptions for drugs of unknown risk. As expected, prescription patterns differed between pregnant and non-pregnant women, favoring drugs with known better safety during gestation among pregnant women (Fig. 2.2). Interestingly however, one in five medications prescribed to pregnant women was considered to be potentially harmful or to have unknown risk. A similar cohort study of prescription medication use in 43,470 pregnant Finnish women revealed that one in five

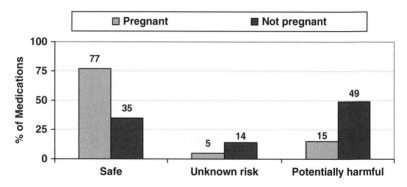

Fig. 2.2 Comparison of prescription risk between pregnant and non-pregnant women (Based on [2])
Pregnancy risk categories were compared for drugs prescribed to pregnant and non-pregnant women. Vitamins, folate, and iron were excluded from this analysis.

similarly purchased at least one drug classified as potentially harmful during pregnancy and 3% purchased at least one drug classified as clearly harmful [3].

> *Pearl for the practitioner:*
> In one large survey, one in five pregnant women was prescribed a potentially harmful medication.

Birth defects affect about 4% of deliveries in the United States, with <1% generally considered to be attributable to maternal drug exposure. Women are often very concerned about medication effects on the developing baby, although the risk, as noted above, is quite low. Clinicians must be able to provide patients with credible information about safe migraine treatment, as unfounded patient fears may result in substantial maternal stress and anxiety and even consideration of pregnancy termination. A negative impact on pregnancy by maternal stress has been supported by studies showing that women exposed to high stress during pregnancy have a higher risk of delivering offspring with low birth weight when babies are born prematurely and a higher incidence of cranial-neural crest malformations (especially cleft lip/palate and conotruncal heart defects [e.g., double-outlet ventricle, tetralogy of Fallot, and ventricular septal defects]) [4,5]. Providing accurate information about safe treatment options can alleviate a considerable amount of the pregnant patient's fear and concern. Since migraine predominates during childbearing years, discussions about the treatment of headaches during pregnancy should ideally occur before conception. Effective planning for treatment during pregnancy helps maximize use of safer therapies and minimize maternal anxiety, excessive headache-related disability, dehydration, and analgesic overuse when standard therapies are excessively restricted.

> **Pearl for the practitioner:**
> Less than 1% of birth defects are attributed to maternal drug exposure. Preconception discussion about real risks and safer treatments reduces patient fears and maximizes focus on the safest therapies.

Understanding Reproductive Risk

Drugs that may result in the development of congenital malformations or other negative fetal outcomes are called teratogens. Negative outcomes may include:

- Altered growth or development;
- Structural malformations;
- Physiological malformations;
- Mortality.

Although teratogen exposure increases the risk of negative fetal outcomes, it does not guarantee the occurrence of any fetal effects. The probability that exposure to a teratogen will result in a negative outcome depends on several factors:

- Drug dosage and duration of exposure;
- Gestational age during exposure;
- Individual susceptibility to exposure;
- Cumulative teratogenic exposures.

Risk of a negative outcome is greater with higher drug dosages and longer duration of exposure, especially when additional use of other teratogenic agents has occurred or the mother or baby are genetically more susceptible to development of a specific malformation or other negative outcome.

Tools for Assessing Reproductive Risk

The most widely used tool for evaluating drug safety during pregnancy in the United States is the Food and Drug Administration (FDA) safety rating system. The FDA system rates medication risk using categories A, B, C, D, and X, based on the available data in human and animal studies (Table 2.1). A survey of FDA pregnancy risk category assignment of drugs in the 2001 and 2002 Physicians' Desk References revealed that >60% of drugs assigned a pregnancy risk category are risk category C (Table 2.2) [6]. While clinicians generally agree that drugs in categories A and B are relatively safe and those in categories D and X should be limited, the majority of medications are classified as the more nebulous category C, reflecting the lack of available risk data for

Table 2.1 FDA risk classification system

Category A: safety established

Controlled studies in women fail to demonstrate a risk to the fetus in the first trimester, there is no evidence of a risk in later trimesters, **AND** the possibility of fetal harm appears remote.

Category B: safety likely

Either animal-reproduction studies have not demonstrated a fetal risk but there are no controlled studies in pregnant women **OR** animal-reproduction studies have shown an adverse effect (other than a decrease in fertility) that was not confirmed in controlled studies in women in the first trimester and there is no evidence of a risk in later trimesters.

Category C: teratogenicity possible

Either studies in animals have revealed adverse effects on the fetus (teratogenic, embryocidal, or other) and there are no controlled studies in women **OR** studies in women and animals are not available. These drugs should be given only if the potential benefit justifies the potential risk to the fetus.

Category D: teratogenicity probable

There is positive evidence of human fetal risk, but the benefits from use in pregnant women may be acceptable despite the risk (e.g., if the drug is needed in a life-threatening situation or for a serious disease for which safer drugs cannot be used or are ineffective).

Category X: teratogenicity likely – contraindicated in pregnancy

Studies in animals and humans have demonstrated fetal abnormalities **AND/OR** there is evidence of fetal risk based on human experience **AND** the risk of the use of the drug in pregnant women clearly outweighs any possible benefit. These drugs are contraindicated in women who are or may become pregnant.

Table 2.2 FDA pregnancy risk categories of drugs in the United States, N (%) (Based on [6])

FDA risk category	2001 PDR $N = 2,249$ drugs	2002 PDR $N = 2,150$ drugs
A	5 (0.2)	7 (0.3)
B	291 (12.9)	296 (13.8)
C	821 (36.5)	802 (37.3)
D	99 (4.4)	81 (3.8)
X	117 (5.2)	124 (5.8)
None listed	916 (40.7)	840 (39.1)

most medications. While FDA pregnancy-risk categories have been a standard for many years, the FDA is currently proposing to eliminate this rating system in favor of providing more detailed sections on pregnancy safety for each drug. Descriptive passages might include more extensive information about what data are available for each drug, detailing whether data are from animal or human studies and contrasting pros and cons of drug exposure. Drug labels will also include a discussion of background risk of specific birth defects to help put warnings into context.

Another source of information is the Teratogen Information System (TERIS), which catalogs risk of teratogenic effects for the offspring of exposed women as none, minimal, small, moderate, or high. When no or limited human data are available, a drug is classified as having an undetermined risk in the TERIS system. An unlikely rating is given when risk is considered to probably be very low, but supportive data are limited.

A comparison of FDA and TERIS risk classifications is shown in Table 2.3. Researchers in the Department of Medical Genetics at the University of British Columbia evaluated drugs approved by the FDA from 1980 to 2000, excluding radioactive agents and drugs subsequently withdrawn from the market [7]. Of the 468 drugs evaluated, a comparison of assigned TERIS ratings to FDA risk category showed a poor correlation. For example, of the 30 drugs identified as having a TERIS risk of none, minimal, or unlikely, 10 received a comparable FDA classification of A or B, while 17 were classified as C and 3 as D or X. This study further highlighted the long period of time that a drug needs to be available on the market before adequate safety data permit determination of risk category. At the time of the study in 2002, 91% of the assessed drugs were still considered to have undetermined pregnancy risk. Two percent of drugs were assigned a TERIS risk designation of small, moderate, or high, with an average time required to identify this risk of 6 years and a range of 3–12 years. Six percent of drugs were assigned a none, minimal, or unlikely TERIS rating, which was determined after an average of 9 years on the market (range of 2–19 years).

Unfortunately, clinicians utilizing several different risk classification systems will soon discover that drugs are not necessarily categorized in comparable risk categories among different systems. For example, pregnancy risk category assignment was compared for drugs common to three different classification systems: the United States FDA, the Australian Drug Evaluation Committee (ADEC), and the Swedish Catalogue of Approved Drugs (FASS) [8]. Only one in four of the drugs common to all three systems received the same risk factor category (Table 2.4). Differences were attributed to disparity in definitions among the three systems, as well as dissimilarities in the way accessible literature was used to determine risk category.

Pearl for the practitioner:
Individual risk classification systems often categorize the safety of drugs differently. Selecting drugs with better safety ratings in several systems can maximize the safety of recommendations.

Table 2.3 Comparison of FDA and TERIS classifications

FDA	TERIS
A, B	None, minimal, or unlikely
C	Undetermined risk
D, X	Small, moderate, or high risk

Table 2.4 Pregnancy risk category assignment for 236 drugs common to three international systems, N (%) (Based on [8])

Risk category	FDA	ADEC	FASS
A	6 (2.5)	50 (21.2)	59 (25.0)
B	62 (26.3)	71 (30.1)	65 (27.2)
C	115 (48.7)	84 (35.6)	85 (36.0)
D	45 (19.1)	29 (12.3)	27 (11.4)
X	8 (3.4)	2 (0.8)	Not used

So what is a clinician to do? While these rating systems certainly have short-comings, the data provided can be used as guides to recommend safer versus less safe alternatives.

Many excellent resources are available that summarize the safety ratings of various drugs to allow the clinician to make more informed recommendations. Patients need to be educated about safety classification options to help determine which specific therapies they will be able to use comfortably. FDA risk categories for specific acute and preventive migraine therapies will be described in detail in Chapters 4 and 6.

> *Pearl for the practitioner:*
> Several safety rating systems are available, but they don't always agree on individual drug safety classifications. Clinicians need to consider inconsistency in rating systems when synthesizing available information to develop relatively safe treatment option recommendations.

Lactation

The American Academy of Pediatrics recommends breastfeeding exclusively during the first 6 months of a baby's life, with additional nursing recommended for at least the baby's first year of life. Breastfeeding has numerous health benefits for the baby (Fig. 2.3):

- Optimizes nutrition;
- Limits exposure to foreign proteins;
- Provides necessary hormones, growth factors, and immune complexes;
- Provides important fatty acids to facilitate good brain development;
- Reduces infant infections and mortality;
- Promotes maternal-baby bonding.

Breastfeeding also benefits the nursing mother [9–11]:

- Assists with return to normal weight;
- Reduces risk for breast cancer;
- Reduces risk for ovarian cancer;

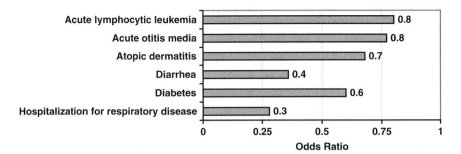

Fig. 2.3 Benefits to developing baby from breastfeeding (Based on [9])
Odds ratios are shown for risk of conditions in term babies who were breast fed compared with those who were bottle fed. Odds ratio for each condition among bottle fed infants was set at 1.0. Data are based on a comprehensive literature review and meta-analyses.

- Reduces risk for rheumatoid arthritis;
- Is cost-effective method of supplying baby's nutrition;
- Improves maternal-baby bonding;
- Delays migraine recurrence during the first postpartum month.

While migraine often disappears or significantly decreases in the second and third trimesters in most pregnant migraineurs, the majority of women will unfortunately experience an unwelcome recurrence of their headaches during the postpartum period. Fortunately, as described in Chapter 1, breastfeeding offers a protective effect against migraine recurrence [11]. Some migraine sufferers may fear unnecessarily that they must either expose their baby to harmful medications to achieve headache control or suffer from untreated, disabling headaches that will negatively impact their ability to care for their new baby. Migraine sufferers may opt to forego breastfeeding due to the fear that nursing will excessively limit their access to effective migraine therapy. Due to the numerous and substantial health benefits for both mother and baby from breastfeeding and the availability of relatively safe therapies, clinicians should encourage women to breastfeed and reassure mothers about the availability of safer, effective treatment options when nursing.

> ***Pearl for the practitioner:***
> Breastfeeding provides important physical and emotional health benefits for both baby and mother. Safer and effective headache treatment options are available for breastfeeding mothers.

Trends in Breastfeeding

National surveys show that 50–90% of women in industrialized countries and >90% in developing countries begin infant nutrition with breastfeeding [12].

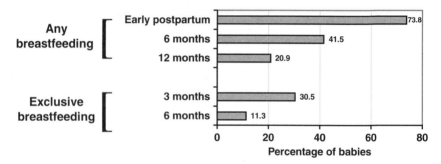

Fig. 2.4 Prevalence of breastfeeding in the United States (Based on [13])
Data are based on a survey of babies born during 2004. Early postpartum refers to the days immediately following delivery and before hospital discharge.

Only about one in three babies worldwide are still breast fed when they are 4 months old. In the United States, most mothers nurse during the first few days of a baby's life, with 2 of every 5 mothers still breastfeeding when the baby is 6 months old and 1 of every 5 mothers breastfeeding when the baby turns 1 year old (Fig. 2.4) [13]. Only one in three mothers exclusively breastfeeds for 3 months. While there may be many reasons women choose not to breastfeed or to discontinue nursing early, safety concerns about headache medications and breastfeeding should be carefully reviewed to ensure the decision to nurse or not is based on sound information.

> *Pearl for the practitioner:*
> Although over half of women breastfeed after delivery, only one in three babies worldwide are still breastfed when they are 4 months old. The decision to not begin or stop breastfeeding early should not be based on the fear that postpartum headaches will go untreated. There are safer, effective treatment options available for women with headaches who choose to breastfeed their infants.

Maternal Drug Effects on the Baby

A variety of factors influence the likelihood that a maternal drug will affect the breastfed baby:

- Timing of drug administration;
- Time to peak drug concentration;
- Drug half-life in both the mother and the baby;
- Drug bioavailability (the amount of medication that enters the blood);
- Factors that influence how much drug appears in breast milk (e.g., molecular weight, as very large drugs are less likely to enter the breast milk).

Formulae exist that can estimate the baby's exposure to drugs in the breast milk [14]. These formulae must consider a wide range of variables:

- Characteristics of the ingested drug, including medication pH and presence of active metabolites;
- Route of administration in the mother;
- Variability in maternal milk composition between and during feedings;
- Variability in infant milk consumption and clearance;
- Age of the baby.

Formula calculations, however, are limited in accurately estimating drug exposure. For example, the initial 10 mL of expressed milk during a feeding has about half of the fat content that will be seen with milk consumed later in the feeding [14]. Consequently, a lower concentration of fat-soluble drugs will be present in the first milk of each feeding. In addition, glomerular filtration and drug metabolism are less robust in younger babies, resulting in lower drug clearance in babies until they are 6–12 months old.

Because of the wide range of patient and pharmacokinetic variables required to accurately measure a baby's true exposure, it is not feasible to calculate risk in most clinical settings individually. In general, risk can be minimized by:

- Selecting drugs with poor transfer into breast milk (e.g., large molecular weight compounds);
- Selecting drugs that are safe in babies;
- Timing maternal drug dosing to minimize exposure in the baby.

Most drugs enter the breast milk through passive diffusion, with transfer highest for fat-soluble drugs. Because milk is slightly more acidic than plasma, basic drugs are more likely to transfer into the breast milk. The milk-to-plasma ratio is a ratio of the level of drug in milk divided by the level of drug in maternal plasma. For example, some migraine medications, such as non-steroidal anti-inflammatory drugs and sumatriptan have a low milk-to-plasma ratio, resulting in minimal effects on the nursing baby. Similarly, the milk-to-plasma ratio is high with topiramate (1.2), while acceptably low with valproic acid (0.42) [15]. The milk-to-plasma ratio is limited, however, by not providing an indication of the absolute drug dose provided by breast milk.

Another method for quantifying the infant exposure through breast milk is the relative infant dose, which is calculated as a percentage of the infant dose to maternal dose [16]. The relative infant dose is calculated by dividing the dose of the drug in milk (mg/kg/day) by the dose administered to the mother each day (mg/kg/day). In term infants, a relative infant dose <10% is generally considered to be safe with short-term use. A lower percentage is preferred for premature babies. A listing of relative infant doses for some medications used in headache treatment is provided in Box 2.1. Consistent with the low milk-to-plasma ratio with non-steroidal anti-inflammatory drugs, naproxen similarly has a low relative infant dose [17]. Among anti-epileptics, topiramate has free passage of drug into breast milk, with high drug

> **Box 2.1** Relative infant dose (generally $<10\%$ is recommended as relatively safe) (Based on [17–20])
>
> - Codeine – 7%
> - Gabapentin – 1–4%
> - Ibuprofen – 0.6%
> - Naproxen – 2–3%
> - Propranolol – 0.2%
> - Sumatriptan – 3–7%
> - Valproic acid – 2%
> - Topiramate – up to 23%

concentrations [18], while relative infant doses are acceptably low with valproic acid (2%) and gabapentin (1–4%) [19,20]. Selecting drugs with lower relative infant doses may also help maximize safety. Recently published data show a lower relative infant dose with sertraline (0.3–0.5%) [21] compared with venlafaxine (6.4%) [19], supporting a preference for sertraline in patients requiring newer antidepressants [22]. Both print and online resources, described below, can help provide extensive information about milk-to-plasma ratios and relative infant doses for a wide variety of medications.

> ***Pearl for the practitioner:***
> Safety of exposure to maternal medications used when nursing can be minimized by selecting drugs with limited concentration in breast milk, drugs that are themselves safe to use in babies, and timing maternal exposure to reduce concentration in milk used for feedings.

Drugs that might affect the baby may still be used by the nursing mother if she and her doctor can identify how long a harmful concentration will be present in her milk following drug ingestion. In general, it is recommended that milk be pumped and dumped for approximately 4 half-lives of the ingested drug to reduce the concentration to safer levels for the baby [23]. For example, if the half-life of a drug is 2 hours, then the mother should pump and discard her milk for 8 hours after medication ingestion. The mother can then supplement the baby with bottle feeding with either stored breast milk or formula during that time. Holding a maternal medication until immediately after nursing may also limit effects on the baby, especially with short-acting acute migraine medications. Furthermore, when baby is sleeping through the night, mother might take her once daily medication immediately after his last feeding before bedtime and possibly dump her first supply of breast milk in the morning.

Published guidance during breastfeeding is available from the American Academy of Pediatrics (AAP), noting drugs that are compatible with breastfeeding and providing citations for reported possible symptoms of concern that require greater caution with use [24]. A brief summary of these guidelines is also available [25]. Several books are regularly updated detailing the latest information on drug safety during nursing, including *Medications and mothers' milk: a manual of lactational pharmacology (medications and mother's milk)* by Thomas W. Hale; and *Drugs in pregnancy and lactation: a reference guide to fetal and neonatal risk (8th edition)* by Gerald G. Briggs, Roger K. Freeman, and Sumner J. Yaffe. Specific recommendations for the use of acute and preventive migraine medications while nursing are provided in Chapters 5 and 7.

Helpful Online and Print Resources

A variety of Internet resources exist that offer information about possible effects of maternal drug exposures, including over-the-counter and prescription medications, herbal products, and illicit drugs (Table 2.5). Reliable books may also be used to help assess the safety of maternal drug use during pregnancy and lactation (Box 2.2). In general, both online and print media utilize widely accepted safety rating systems, such as the FDA, TERIS, and AAP classification systems, supplemented by additional reviews of available literature and results of clinical practice experiences.

Box 2.2 Print resources

- *Drugs during pregnancy and lactation*, by Christ of Schaefer, Paul W. Peters, and Richard K Miller, published by Academic Press, 2007
- *Medications and mothers' milk: a manual of lactational pharmacology (medications and mother's milk)*, by Thomas W. Hale, published by Pharmasoft Medical Publishing, 2008
- *Drugs in pregnancy and lactation: a reference guide to fetal and neonatal risk (8th edition)*, by Gerald G. Briggs, Roger K Freeman, and Sumner J Yaffe, published by Lippincott Williams & Wilkins, 2008
- *Medication safety in pregnancy and breastfeeding*, by Gideon Koren, published by McGraw-Hill, 2007
- *Textbook of human lactation*, by Thomas W. Hale and Peter E. Hartmann, published by Hale Hartmann's, 2007.

Table 2.5 Internet resources for medication use during pregnancy and lactation

Website	Site Sponsor	Information Available
Pregnancy information		
http://otispregnancy.org/	Organization of Teratology Information Services	Free fact sheets available for a range of treatments. Available migraine drugs include: acetaminophen, antidepressants, caffeine, & St. John's wort
http://www.reprotox.org/.	Reproductive Toxicology Center	Membership provides access to information for a wide range of therapies, with detailed references provided for each compound.
http://depts.washington.edu/terisweb/teris/	Teratogen Information System (TERIS)	Subscription provides TERIS summaries of drugs, including quantification of both level of risk and quality of data analyzed. Online version of *Shepard's Catalog of Teratogenic Agents* is also available.
http://www.safefetus.com/	King's College London	Provides FDA recommendations for the use of medications during pregnancy and breastfeeding (when available).
http://www.motherisk.com	The Hospital for Sick Children of the University of Toronto	Evidence-based information on drug safety during pregnancy and breastfeeding

Table 2.5 (continued)

Website	Site Sponsor	Information Available
Lactation information		
http://www.babycenter.com/0_drug-safety-during-breastfeeding_8790.bc?Ad=com.bc.common.AdInfo_401a60ca44	Recommendations developed by pharmacist and director of Drug Information Service at University of California, San Diego	Wide assortment of commonly used prescription and non-prescription medications divided into 4 categories: safe, probably safe, potentially hazardous, and not safe
http://neonatal.ttuhsc.edu/lact/	Thomas W. Hale, RPh, PhD, Professor of Pediatrics at Texas Tech University	In addition to a huge listing of therapies for which safety information is provided, healthcare providers can post questions directly to Dr. Hale.
http://www.breastfeedingbasics.com/html/drugs_and_bf.shtml	Anne Smith, BA, an international board-certified lactation consultant	Comprehensive overview of drug use with breastfeeding with information appropriate for both clinician and patient
http://www.motherisk.com	The Hospital for Sick Children of the University of Toronto	Evidence-based information on drug safety during pregnancy and breastfeeding

Summary

Information on the safety of medications during pregnancy and lactation is generally derived from cohort and case-controlled studies. Despite limitations in available safety data, widely accepted drug safety rating systems, like the FDA risk classification and TERIS systems, provide a synthesis of available data to help develop rational therapeutic recommendations. Fortunately, medication-related birth defects are very rare and selecting drugs generally considered to be safe or relatively safe can minimize risks. The baby's safety from exposure to medications used by the nursing mother can be estimated by understanding the characteristics of the drug and the timing of exposure. Using information from available rating systems and other resources allows the clinician to offer knowledgeable recommendations for safer treatments during pregnancy and lactation.

Practical pointers:

- Although women often state a desire to avoid medications during pregnancy, almost all women will use over-the-counter drugs. Nearly 2/3 will use prescriptions and almost half will take herbal remedies.
- Medication-related birth defects occur rarely.
- Several, well-accepted systems are available to categorize drug safety, although disagreement on individual drug safety ratings often occurs when comparing ratings for the same drug in various systems.
- Many factors affect the safety for the baby from medication ingested by the breastfeeding mother. Published guidelines account for these factors when making recommendations.

References

1. Glover DD, Amonkar M, Rybeck BF, Tracy TS. Prescription, over-the-counter, and herbal medicine use in a rural, obstetric population. *Am J Obstet Gynecol* 2003;188:1039–1045.
2. Schirm E, Meijer WM, Tobi H, de Jong-van den Berg LW. Drug use by pregnant women and comparable non-pregnant women in the Netherlands with reference to the Australian classification system. *Eur J Obstet Gynecol Reprod Biol* 2004;114:182–188.
3. Malm H, Martikainen J, Klaukka T, Neuvonen PJ. Prescription of hazardous drugs during pregnancy. *Drug Saf* 2004;27:889–908.
4. Precht DH, Andersen PK, Olsen J. Severe life events and impaired fetal growth: a nationwide study with complete follow-up. *Acta Obstet Gynecol Scand* 2007;86:266–275.
5. Hansen D, Lou HC, Olsen J. Serious life events and congenital malformations: a national study with complete follow-up. *Lancet* 2000;356:875–880.
6. Uhl K, Kennedy DL, Kweder SL. Risk management strategies in the Physicians' Desk Reference product labels for pregnancy category X drugs. *Drug Saf* 2002;25:885–892.

7. Lo WY, Firedman JM. Teratogenicity of recently introduced medications in human pregnancy. *Obstet Gynecol* 2002;100:465–473.
8. Addis A, Sharabi S, Bonati M. Risk classification systems for drug use during pregnancy. Are they a reliable source of information? *Drug Saf* 2000;23:245–253.
9. Ip S, Chung M, Raman G, et al. Breastfeeding and maternal and infant health outcomes in developed countries. *Evid Rep Technol Assess (Full Rep)* 2007;135:1–186.
10. Pikwer M, Bergström U, Nilsson JA, et al. Breast-feeding, but not oral contraceptives, is associated with a reduced risk of rheumatoid arthritis. *Ann Rheum Dis*, in press.
11. Sances G, Granella F, Nappi RE, et al. Course of migraine during pregnancy and postpartum: a prospective study. *Cephalalgia* 2003;23:197–205.
12. Heird WC. Progress in promoting breast-feeding, combating malnutrition, and composition and use of infant formula, 1981–2006. *J Nutr* 2007;137:499S–502S.
13. Centers for Disease Control and Prevention. Breastfeeding trends and updated national health objectives for exclusive breastfeeding – United States, birth years 2000–2004. *Morb Mortal Wkly Rep* 2007;56:760–763.
14. McNamara PJ, Abbassi M. Neonatal exposure to drugs in breast milk. *Pharma Res* 2004;21:555–566.
15. Dharamsi A, Smith J. Drugs in breast milk 2003, 6th edition. Clinical Pharmacy Bulletin, available at http://www.cw.bc.ca/newborncare/pdf-clinical/DrugsInBreastMilk.pdf. Accessed July 2008.
16. Lee KG. Lactation and drugs. *Paediatrics Child Health* 2007;17:68–71.
17. Matheson I, Kristensen K, Lunde PM. Drug utilization in breast-feeding women. A survey in Oslo. *Eur J Clin Pharmacol* 1990;38:453–459.
18. Hale TW. Drug therapy and breastfeeding: antibiotics, analgesics, and other medications. *NeoReviews* 2005;6:e233.
19. Ostrea EM, Mantaring JB, Silvestre MA. Drugs that affect the fetus and newborn infant via the placenta or breast milk. *Pediatr Clin N Am* 2004;51:539–579.
20. Kristensen JH, Ilett KF, Hackett P, Kohan R. Gabapentin and breastfeeding: a case report. *J Hum Lact* 2006;22:426.
21. http://apps.cignabehavioral.com/web/basicsite/provider/treatingBehavioralConditions/PsychotropicMedicationDuringPregnancy.pdf. Accessed July 2008.
22. Therapeutic Guidelines Limited, amended February 2007. Available at http://www.tg.com.au/etg_demo/tgc/plg/5a57cf7.htm. Accessed July 2008.
23. http://www.medsafe.govt.nz/Profs/PUarticles/lactation.htm. Accessed May 2008.
24. American Academy of Pediatric Committee on Drugs. The transfer of drugs and other chemicals into human milk. *Pediatrics* 2001;108:776–789.
25. Ressel G. AAP updates statement for transfer of drugs and other chemicals into breast milk. *Am Fam Physician* 2002;65:979–980.

Chapter 3
Non-Pharmacological Headache Treatments

Key Chapter Points

- Non-drug headache treatments that can be safely used during pregnancy and lactation include pain management techniques, exercise, smoking cessation, and lifestyle regulation.
- Non-pharmacological approaches can be helpful during preconception, pregnancy, and lactation.
- Relaxation and stress management are the most effective non-drug treatments.
- Dietary recommendations during pregnancy and lactation include not skipping meals, consuming regular, nutritious, balanced meals and snacks, maintaining adequate hydration, and using prenatal vitamins. Elimination diets are usually not helpful and should not be recommended during pregnancy.
- Other useful modalities include aerobic exercise, physical therapy, and massage.

Keywords Biofeedback · Diet · Exercise · Oral splint · Relaxation · Trigger

When my headache starts, I tell the kids they have to go to their rooms for quiet reading, while I retreat to my bedroom. I turn off the lights, unplug anything that makes a sound, and put a washcloth over my eyes to make sure it's totally dark. Then I lie in bed and wait for my headache to inevitably get worse. My mom always did the same thing. Now that I'm pregnant, I don't want to take any medicine, so I guess I'll just suffer like mom did.

Patients often develop a negative, catastrophizing attitude about their headaches, especially after they become pregnant. Women may incorrectly assume that few effective treatments are available when pregnant and nursing. Fortunately, non-drug headache treatments can be very effective and are not equivalent to "just toughing it out" in hopeless isolation. Ideally, patients should receive instruction for these techniques prior to conception, when they can continue to use their standard headache rescue therapy while mastering non-pharmacological skills. Non-drug treatment options are complementary to

D.A. Marcus, P.A. Bain, *Effective Migraine Treatment in Pregnant and Lactating Women: A Practical Guide*, DOI 10.1007/978-1-60327-439-5_3, © Humana Press, a part of Springer Science+Business Media, LLC 2009

pharmacologic options, and developing effective use of non-pharmacologic therapies can help reduce requirements for medications to treat headache pain during pregnancy and when breastfeeding.

Non-pharmacologic therapies reduce headache activity by reducing exposure or response to headache triggers and/or altering brain levels of pain-provoking neurochemicals. Headache triggers can sometimes be avoided (e.g., eating regular meals to avoid fasting) or the body's natural physiological response to triggers can be modified (e.g., learning stress management). Some techniques help block pain signal transmission by altering serotonin levels (e.g., relaxation or biofeedback can alter the metabolism of serotonin) or muscle tension (e.g., myofascial techniques and exercise). Healthy lifestyle habits (e.g., eating regular meals, achieving adequate sleep, avoiding nicotine, and practicing stress management) can reduce muscle tension, decrease pain, and improve functional status. Pain management skills, such as relaxation, biofeedback, and stress management, are particularly effective, easy-to-learn strategies to help minimize headaches. These treatments function primarily as headache preventive therapies, although relaxation and biofeedback, exercises, and heat or ice application may also be used to reduce the severity of acute headache episodes.

> *Pearl for the practitioner:*
> Non-drug treatments reduce headache by restricting exposure to modifiable triggers, altering the body's physiological response to triggers and stress, or changing levels of pain-provoking neurochemicals, like serotonin.

Even without specific training, patients often utilize pain-relieving, non-drug behaviors to reduce headache severity. In one study, consecutive patients with migraine ($N = 75$) or tension-type ($N = 55$) headaches were asked about their behaviors during a headache and "tricks" they used to relieve their pain (Fig. 3.1) [1]. Many of these tricks and behaviors have been found to be effective by trial and error. Encouraging patients to engage in helpful behaviors reinforces the active role that patients should play in helping to control their headaches and headache-related disability.

Educating patients about their headaches and effective therapies (both drug and non-drug options) substantially increases the success of headache treatment. In a recent study, 100 consecutive migraine patients were randomly assigned to usual medical care or usual care plus three educational classes on headache pathogenesis and pain management techniques. The classes were taught by trained lay instructors. After six months, those patients who had been exposed to the additional education experienced significantly reduced migraine-related disability ($P<0.05$), as well as greater reductions in headache frequency (Fig. 3.2) [2].

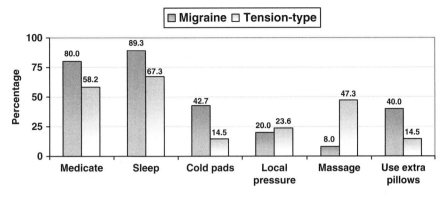

Fig. 3.1 Patient responses to headache (Based on [1])

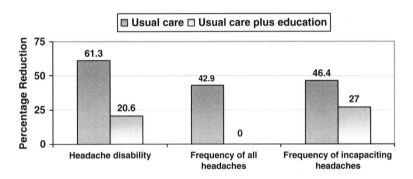

Fig. 3.2 Benefit of headache education (Based on [2])

Patients do not need to choose between medication and non-medication treatments, because they are usually complementary. For example, the addition of biofeedback to standard migraine preventive therapy improves the benefit to greater than that seen with either treatment alone [3]. During pregnancy, patients should focus primarily on safer, non-drug treatments, reserving medications for more recalcitrant headaches. This chapter will describe those treatments that have shown the strongest efficacy for headache relief. Patient instructional handouts describing specific non-drug techniques are provided in Chapter 10.

Pearl for the practitioner:
Non-drug options complement medication headache treatments.

Trigger Identification and Avoidance

Patients frequently report a variety of internal and external triggers that cause increased headache activity. Common triggers include the internal trigger of hormonal changes and external triggers of stress, glare, skipped meals, noise, and sleep disruption. Stress is the most common trigger (75%), with menses, odors, sleep irregularities, weather, fasting, and exertion as the next most commonly listed triggers [4]. Although most patients endorse triggers at least occasionally provoking a headache, consistent triggers are less common. In a survey of 1,750 consecutive migraine patients, 76% of patients endorsed having migraine triggers, although most triggers produced a headache only occasionally (Table 3.1) [5].

Cause or Coincidence?

Although patients may note the occurrence of headache after trigger exposure, this relationship does not necessarily confirm a cause and effect. Few triggers have or can be conclusively proven to consistently be related to headache provocation. In an interesting provocative study, 68 headache sufferers (ages 18–30 years old) experiencing at least one headache weekly for at least the preceding six months were exposed to stress or noise, with subsequent headache activity monitored [6]. Stress was induced by asking the subjects to solve difficult anagrams, and then providing feedback that they had failed to solve the puzzles. Noise consisted of 50 dB white noise. Both triggers effectively provoked headaches, supporting patients' reports that stress and noise

Table 3.1 Common migraine triggers (Based on [5])

Trigger	Provokes >1/3 headaches (% patients)	Provokes >2/3 headaches (% patients)
Stress	79.7	25.5
Hormones	65.1	33.3
Fasting/skipping meals	57.3	12.0
Weather	53.2	11.3
Sleep disturbance	49.8	8.6
Odor	43.7	10.7
Neck pain	38.4	10.6
Lights	38.1	6.9
Alcohol	37.8	9.5
Smoke	35.7	6.9
Sleeping late	32.0	4.4
Heat	30.3	5.4
Food	26.9	4.3
Exercise	22.1	2.2
Sex	5.2	0.3

exposure can induce their headaches. These data also confirm recommendations to minimize stress and external stimulation from noise to reduce disability associated with headache attacks.

Several studies have attempted to correlate the ingestion of specific foods and subsequent headache activity. Putative headache triggers include food items that are rich in proteins known to affect vascular activity, such as foods containing tyramine (aged cheeses, alcohol, sour cream), phenylethylamine (chocolate), nitrates (hot dogs), and dopamine (broad bean pods). One study compared headache activity in a group of migraineurs when eating their usual diet compared with two structured diets: one diet required high consumption of alleged headache trigger foods, while the other diet restricted these same foods [7]. Headache improved similarly when following either structured diet, with headache activity generally unrelated to specific food ingestion. Headaches, however, did seem to occur more frequently when patients had been fasting, drank alcohol, or ate chocolate. Restricting foods containing tyramine, nitrates, and dopamine was not helpful, suggesting a limited role for dietary elimination in headache management.

Two studies have evaluated headache relationship to individual food ingestion. One study showed that large daily doses of aspartame (Nutrasweet®) for four weeks increased headache frequency but not severity in migraineurs who previously reported that aspartame was a headache trigger [8]. Study participants ingested very large doses of aspartame (300 mg) four times a day. This is the equivalent of drinking 12 cans of diet soda or ingesting 32 packets of sweetener everyday for a month. More moderate use was not tested; however, this study showed only a small increase in headache after regularly eating very large amounts of aspartame. A second study directly tested chocolate ingestion as a trigger in 63 women with chronic headaches by asking the women to follow a restrictive diet eliminating typical putative headache trigger foods and then consume 60 g chocolate-flavored bars on 4 occasions, with headache activity measured before and after consumption [9]. Two of these bars were chocolate and two were carob, which does not contain presumed trigger chemicals. All samples were flavored with mint to prevent identifying which bars were the actual chocolate bars. Even women who reported they believed chocolate triggered their headaches did not have headaches triggered when they didn't know if they were eating actual chocolate or the carob placebo. Cheating on the diet and eating other restrictive foods like peanut butter, colas, or pizza along with chocolate did not result in increased headache activity either. Summarizing these data, it appears that restrictive or elimination diets have limited impact on headache patterns.

Pearl for the practitioner:
Restricting all presumed headache food triggers is unlikely to be helpful in reducing headache frequency or severity for most patients. It is more prudent to provide resources detailing common triggers and ask the patient to pay particular attention to those select triggers that consistently bring on headaches.

Dietary Recommendations During Pregnancy and Lactation

Patients should be informed that elimination diets typically don't reduce headaches, while eating regular meals and a balanced healthy diet can improve headache activity. Since individual foods rarely seem to trigger headache, why are there such strong myths about them as headache triggers? About one in three migraine sufferers will report warning symptoms of an impending headache occurring several hours or even a couple of days before the onset of head pain, called a migraine prodrome [10]. Prodromal symptoms often include fatigue, mood disturbance, and gastrointestinal symptoms. Food craving may also occur as part of this prodrome, causing a false association between eating the food and getting a headache. The food ingestion doesn't actually trigger the headache, but is a sign that the headache process has already begun. In addition, craving sweets typically occurs in response to stress, fasting, and menses. Therefore, the actual headache trigger might be the stress, fasting, or hormonal changes, while subsequent chocolate ingestion is actually a reaction to the trigger rather than acting as a provoking factor itself.

> **Pearl for the practitioner:**
> Strict elimination diets are usually not helpful and may be harmful in pregnant and/or breastfeeding patients because they may result in decreasing important intake of nutritious foods at a time when proper nutrition is essential. The most beneficial headache dietary advice is to not skip meals and avoid becoming dehydrated.

Trigger Avoidance or Desensitization?

Many possible headache triggers, such as change in the weather or exposure to life stresses, are impossible to avoid. Others, such as foods, wine, noise, and glare, may be easier to eliminate. In an interesting series of experiments, Martin and colleagues in Australia evaluated the effects of short- and long-duration exposure to a variety of possible headache triggers, including flickering lights, noise, and stress [11–13]. While short-duration exposure increased headache activity, long-duration exposure seemed to reduce pain ratings by desensitizing patients to the effects of subsequent short-duration exposure. These data suggest that headache sufferers may become less sensitive and responsive to triggers if repeatedly exposed to low levels of a trigger, using levels that would be inadequate to provoke a headache attack. These researchers questioned the conventional wisdom of prescribing trigger avoidance, suggesting that successful avoidance of commonly encountered triggers might increase the provocation response when exposure inevitably occurs.

These data support skill training to reduce a negative physiological response when exposed to triggers rather than primarily focusing on trigger avoidance. This approach may be particularly beneficial for triggers that truly cannot be avoided, like stress. Therefore, patients should be counseled to limit exposure to those triggers they might successfully avoid (like fasting). However, suggesting excessive restrictions in exposure to stimulation, such as prolonged use of sunglasses, light dimming, and noise reduction, may actually increase patients' responses to these triggers for future headaches.

> *Pearl for the practitioner:*
> Exposure to low levels of trigger factors that cannot be entirely avoided may help desensitize patients to their headache-triggering effects. Excessive stimulation restriction between headache episodes may in fact make the patient more sensitive to headache provocation when inevitably exposed to that trigger.

Psychological Pain Management Skills

The most effective headache-reducing non-drug treatments are pain management skills. Although often called psychological skills, benefit from these skills does not imply that the headaches are psychologically-based. These skills work by teaching the brain to activate natural pain-relieving mechanisms while suppressing pain-signaling pathways. Psychological techniques teach the brain to distract itself from headache messages by focusing on non-pain signals. Patient instructional sheets for psychological pain management skills are provided in Chapter 10 and on the accompanying CD.

Relaxation and Biofeedback

Relaxation techniques, including biofeedback, are among the most effective preventive therapies for migraine and tension-type headaches. Relaxation techniques can include visual imagery, deep breathing techniques, and progressive muscle relaxation. Biofeedback is a type of relaxation that relies on external biological parameters (e.g., finger temperature, respiratory rate, and muscle tone) to provide objective data of a relaxation state before and after intervention. Biofeedback can include complex computerized monitors of muscle contraction with graphic displays to provide feedback to the patient, or simple hand-held thermometers designed to demonstrate a few degree increase in hand temperature when relaxation has been achieved (to about 96 degrees Fahrenheit or 35–36 degrees Celsius). An inexpensive hand-held thermometer and biofeedback recording can be obtained from Primary Care Network at 800-769-7565.

More expensive digital biofeedback monitors can be purchased from several companies (available on the Internet) for about 20 dollars. No single relaxation technique is superior to the others, although some patients find that they prefer using one technique over another. In general, biofeedback can be taught by a trained therapist over about five or six treatment sessions, with patients practicing techniques at home between sessions. Once patients have mastered these skills, they no longer have to use them regularly, but may use them as needed.

The success of these techniques may result in a false perception that headache sufferers are merely nervous people and that their headaches will go away if they "chill out." Research confirms that these techniques actually change levels of important pain neurochemicals, such as serotonin, in a similar way to those changes seen with the use of headache preventive therapies, like the antidepressants [14]. Training in relaxation or biofeedback can result in changes in the metabolism of serotonin that will result in improved headache control. The feeling related to achieving a state of relaxation, relaxed muscles, or warmed hand temperature is a signal that the appropriate pain-relieving pathways have been activated within the nervous system.

Relaxation or biofeedback techniques have similar efficacy to standard migraine preventive medications, without associated side effects. About 50–80% of patients motivated to learn these techniques experience relief [15–17]. In a recent study, benefits from six months' training with relaxation and biofeedback versus propranolol were compared in 192 migraine patients [17]. Headache frequency, duration, and severity were significantly improved with either treatment ($P<0.05$), with no between-group differences (Fig. 3.3). After completing 6 months of treatment, home practice with relaxation and biofeedback and propranolol were both tapered to off. Headache resurgence was defined as an increase in headache activity of at least 50%. Return of headaches was significantly more frequent among patients treated with propranolol ($P<0.001$), demonstrating a superior long-term prophylactic effect with non-drug therapy.

Relaxation During Pregnancy and Lactation

Relaxation and biofeedback have been specifically tested during pregnancy and lactation. A controlled clinical trial demonstrated both short- and long-term efficacy from relaxation with thermal biofeedback during pregnancy [18,19]. Significant headache reduction occurred for 73% treated with biofeedback versus 29% assigned to an attention control, where research subjects spent similar time with a therapist but were not trained in any pain-relieving skills [18]. Benefits were maintained up to one year postpartum in 68% of treated subjects [19].

> **Pearl for the practitioner:**
> Relaxation and biofeedback effectively reduce headaches during pregnancy and breastfeeding for two-thirds of women learning these techniques.

A. Relaxation with biofeedback (N = 96)

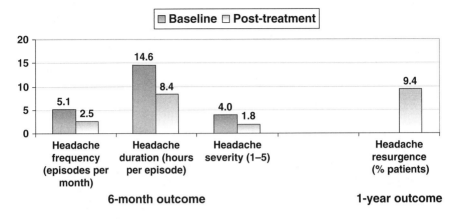

B. Propranolol 80 mg daily (N = 96)

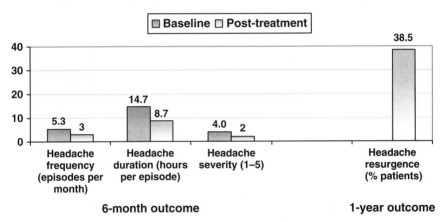

Fig. 3.3 Six-month headache improvement with biofeedback vs. propranolol (Based on [17])
Headache severity was rated on a 5-point scale from 1 (mild) to 5 (severe). After 6 months, home practice with relaxation and biofeedback and propranolol were both tapered to off. Headache resurgence was defined as an increase in headache activity of at least 50%.

Stress Management

Stress is the most commonly reported headache trigger. Stress may also be an important factor in the development of new headaches. In an interesting recent study, incident headache was evaluated, based on exposure to work stress, as measured by a high work-effort to work-reward imbalance. High work stress resulted in a 26% increased risk for developing new onset migraine [20].

Exposure to stress results in painful muscle contraction, as well as changes in pain chemicals in the nervous system, such as serotonin [21], endorphins [22], norepinephrine, and dopamine [23], that lead to increased headache suscept-ibility. The occurrence of life stressors is related to both headache frequency and severity [24]. Stress management is not a recommendation to eliminate exposure to stressful situations. Everyone's life is full of stress, including minor stresses, like confronting traffic or waiting in line at the store, and major stresses, like moving, having children, or facing the death of a loved one. While exposure to these stresses cannot be eliminated, patients can learn to change their body's physiological response when encountering stress.

> **Pearl for the practitioner:**
> Stress is the most common headache trigger. Stress management reduces headaches by changing the body's physiological response to stress expo-sure. While the sources of the stress often cannot be changed, one can change her reaction to the stress.

Stress management results in improvement in migraine by about 60% [25,26]. The effectiveness of an eight-week home-based stress management program was compared with treatment with standard doses of amitriptyline [27]. Improvement in headache activity and reduction in medication use occurred for both groups, with superior reduction with stress management training (58% reduction) versus amitriptyline (33% reduction). In addition, the stress man-agement group had an increase in their internal locus of control, the perception that the patient has the ability to control her own headaches rather than head-aches being controlled by fate or healthcare providers.

Cognitive Restructuring

Cognitive restructuring describes a change in thoughts from negative to posi-tive. For example, most patients with chronic pain experience times when pain levels increase or flare, possibly related to an activity or for unknown reasons. Negative thoughts about the pain include catastrophic thinking that the pain will never improve, that nothing the patient does ever helps, and that achieving pain relief is hopeless. More positive self-messages would include thoughts about how pain management skills can help reduce their pain, that the pain will improve, and that they can change their behavior (e.g., taking more breaks during an activity) to reduce future pain flares.

Patients should be counseled about reasonable expectations for their head-aches. Unreasonable expectations include thinking that they should never experience another headache or that medication alone will always be enough to keep pain under control. Even with effective pain management, most patients with chronic headaches will continue to experience at least some headaches, even during pregnancy. Realistic goals include decreased:

- Headache severity;
- Headache frequency;
- Headache duration;
- Interference from headaches;
- Reliance on medications.

Patients should be encouraged to actively treat their headaches with positive behaviors like relaxation techniques, aerobic exercise, stretching, ice packs, etc. rather than passive behaviors like retreating to a dark quiet room and lying in bed. While trigger avoidance and stimulus control (e.g., seeking isolation from external stimulation) may be necessary for very severe episodes, active behaviors can provide important distractions during milder attacks to prevent escalation to more severe and incapacitating headaches. Developing a sense that one can positively affect one's fate results in a more positive sense of self-control. This development of self-efficacy or a sense of personal locus of control over pain management has been linked to decreased headache-associated disability [28].

> *Pearls for the practitioner:*
> Patients will improve control over their headaches if they develop realistic goals for headache management, positive self-messages about headache, and active behaviors when pain begins. Healthcare providers should help patients feel that the patient has the ability to control her headaches.

Distraction

The brain can only focus on so many things at once. For example, it's hard to balance your checkbook when your toddler is running around the room, your teenager is negotiating for more time with the family car, and the television is blaring in the other room. Patients often find, particularly when their headache is mild, that they can reduce their perception of pain signals by distracting the brain with other, non-pain messages.

Historically, headache sufferers have often been encouraged to retreat to a dark, quiet room with their headache. While this becomes necessary when the headache is very severe (such as when vomiting has occurred), isolation typically intensifies milder headaches. Strict stimulus control can decrease aggravating headache triggers; however, the headache sufferer also loses distractions from the pain signals, generally leading to a greater focus on discomfort and increased symptom severity. Consequently, unless the headache symptoms are very severe, patients should be encouraged to engage in pleasant, distracting behaviors when a headache first begins:

- Going outside for a brisk walk or gentle swim;
- Listening to soothing music;
- Performing stretching exercises;
- Using relaxation techniques;
- Applying ice to the neck.

While these distracting behaviors will not necessarily control every headache, they can help maintain function, reduce focusing on headache symptoms, and decrease the likelihood of pain escalation. Consistently utilizing these techniques helps the patient gain a sense of personal control over her headaches, shifting the locus of control from fate or healthcare providers to the patient herself.

Pearl for the practitioner:
For most headache episodes, patients should be encouraged to utilize positive, active behaviors to maintain a sense of control and provide distractions from pain. Withdrawal behaviors and strict stimulus control should be reserved for the most severe, disabling headache episodes.

Effective Psychological Pain Management Technique Delivery Systems

Psychological pain management skills can be effectively taught through a wide variety of delivery systems in individualized or group settings (Box 3.1). Costs from individualized treatment can be limited by using a minimal therapist approach, which relies on consistent patient home training and practice between therapy appointments. Recently, benefit has also been demonstrated by using migraine patients trained to teach non-pharmacologic therapies to fellow patients, although benefits were more modest compared to studies using professionals as instructors [29].

Box 3.1 Effective delivery methods for psychological pain management skills

- Individualized therapy, including minimal therapist contact approach
- Group therapy
- Lay trainer
- Remote learning
  - Written materials
  - Internet-based treatment
  - Telephone instructions

Patients with limited access to psychological services can also effectively learn relaxation and stress management techniques through online training and other educational resources. Studies have shown benefit when psychological management techniques are taught using home training with written materials [30], telephone-administered therapy [31], or Internet-based education [32].

> *Pearl for the practitioner:*
> Psychological headache-relieving therapies can be taught using therapists, trained lay instructors, and/or self-help resources.

Healthy Lifestyle Habits

Diet

Nutritional needs increase during pregnancy and lactation and women should be strongly encouraged to achieve adequate nutrition through eating regular, well-balanced meals and snacks throughout the day. Dietary restrictions, such as following a tyramine-free diet, are probably beneficial for only about one in three migraineurs and, as described above, are not recommended during pregnancy and lactation because they may unnecessarily restrict nutritious foods, such as calcium-rich dairy foods and vitamin-rich fruits and vegetables. While consuming specific foods is usually not linked to headache exacerbation, fasting has consistently been shown to aggravate headache and should be avoided by consuming regular meals [33–35].

> *Pearl for the practitioner:*
> Skipping meals is a potent headache trigger. Pregnant and breastfeeding women should be encouraged to eat regularly.

Pregnant and nursing mothers should also be counseled to achieve adequate hydration. In general, individuals need to drink 1–1.5 liters of water for every 1000 calories consumed, so a person eating a 2000-calorie diet will need to drink 2–3 liters of water daily [36]. Since pregnant women need to increase their caloric intake by about 300 calories in general during the second trimester, they should consume an additional half-liter of water daily. In general, women are recommended to drink 8–10 glasses of water daily during pregnancy [36]. During breastfeeding, women are advised to drink one glass of water with each meal plus a glass of water every time they nurse [36]. Adequate hydration may also reduce headaches. In a small pilot study, increasing daily fluid intake in non-pregnant patients by one liter daily resulted in modest reductions in headache activity [37].

Pearl for the practitioner:
Adequate hydration is important during pregnancy and breastfeeding. These women should be encouraged to drink 8–10 glasses of water daily.

Supplementation with prenatal vitamins and folate should be encouraged in all pregnant women to achieve adequate nutrient intake, particularly if headache activity is limiting food intake. A recent meta-analysis demonstrated consistent and significant reductions in the occurrence of neural tube, cardiovascular, and limb defects in the offspring of women using prenatal vitamins with folate [38]. The Centers for Disease Control (CDC) and other public health organizations recommend that all women capable of becoming pregnant should consume 0.4 mg of folic acid daily [39]. This can be achieved by diets that include folate-enriched bread, cereal, rice, or pasta; lentils, legumes, leafy green vegetables, and citrus fruits; or by the use of a vitamin supplement. From the available evidence, the CDC has estimated that as many as 50% of the cases of neural tube defects could be avoided with folate supplementation [40].

Pearl for the practitioner:
Women of child-bearing potential should consume 0.4 mg (400 micrograms) of folic acid daily to minimize risk for neural tube defects.

Sleep

Sleep disturbances have been consistently linked to increased migraine activity. At a tertiary headache center, change in sleep was endorsed as usually triggering a headache for 26% of almost 300 consecutive headache patients [41]. In a second, larger sample of migraine patients ($N = 1283$), sleep disturbance was similarly reported to be a frequent migraine trigger in 27% [52]. Additionally, 14% identified sleeping late as a frequent headache trigger.

Physiology of Sleep and Headache

Circulating tryptophan is converted to serotonin in the pineal gland; pineal serotonin is then converted to melatonin at night [42]. Serotonin and melatonin released from the pineal gland influence activity of the trigeminovascular system, suggesting a possible link with migraine. Interestingly, plasma melatonin levels drawn at 11:00 PM were significantly higher in 93 migraineurs compared with 46 age-matched controls (33 vs. 52 pg/ml, $P<0.001$) [43]. It has been postulated that elevated pineal serotonin and reduced melatonin will increase headache activity through the trigeminovascular system [42].

In addition to possible roles for changes in serotonin and melatonin in influencing a migraine-sleep link, magnesium deficiency has long been postulated to play an important role in the development of acute migraine episodes [44–46]. Magnesium balance has also been hypothesized to relate to biorhythms via the pineal gland [47]. Higher magnesium levels in the brain have been linked to improved sleep quality in experimental mice [48]. A small study evaluating cardiac and autonomic effects of chronic sleep deprivation in 30 healthy male college students found a small but significant reduction in intracellular magnesium (5.6 to 5.2 mg/dL, $P<0.05$) [49]. A direct relationship between this reduction in magnesium from poor sleep and increased migraine activity has not been studied.

Effect of Sleep Disturbance on Headache

Patient reports of sleep disturbance have been consistently linked with increased headache activity. Information about sleep disturbance during the preceding three months was gathered in 2,662 general practice patients, showing that headache sufferers were more likely to report mild (odds ratio 2.4), moderate (odds ratio 3.6), or severe sleep disturbances (odds ratio 7.5) [50]. Furthermore, sleep disturbance was more likely in patients with more frequent or more severe headaches. A similar comparison identified poor sleep in 64% of migraineurs versus 33% of controls [51]. The most notable difference was significantly longer sleep latency in migraineurs compared with controls (25 vs. 10 minutes, $P<0.01$).

Another survey of 1,283 migraine patients identified frequent trouble with falling asleep in 31%, staying asleep in 39%, and insomnia (sleeping ≤ 6 hours nightly) in 38% [52]. Insomnia would have been expected to occur in 11% of an analogous general population sample. Furthermore, in this study, routine sleep duration was correlated with headache activity. Mean number of headaches per month was greater in migraineurs routinely sleeping ≤ 6 hours nightly (17.6 headaches) or >8 hours nightly (17.5 headaches) compared with normal sleep (15.1 headaches). Severe headache days per month were similarly higher for patients with insufficient (7.3 severe headache days) and excessive sleep (6.6 severe headache days) compared with migraineurs reporting normal sleep (5.9 severe headache days). These differences reached statistical significance for the insufficient sleep group ($P<0.01$). Differences were not statistically significant for the excessive sleep group, likely due to a relatively small number of patients in this sample ($N=73$).

Sleep and Pregnancy

Data from the studies reported above suggest that headache sufferers should be encouraged to consistently sleep more than 6 hours and up to 8 hours nightly. Although studies have not specifically tested the effect of improved sleep on headache activity, 69–89% of migraineurs and 67% of tension-type patients report using sleep therapeutically for acute headaches [52].

> *Pearl for the practitioner:*
> Improved sleep has been linked to reduced headache activity. Women should be advised to sleep between 6 and 8 hours nightly. Many non-drug sleep hygiene recommendations can help to improve sleep.

Regulating sleep may be particularly beneficial for pregnant women, who are more likely to report sleep disturbances. A prospective survey of 325 women compared sleep patterns before pregnancy and during each trimester [53]. The following patterns were recorded pre-pregnancy and during the 1st, 2nd, and 3rd trimesters, respectively: total sleep 8.0, 8.7, 8.4, and 8.3 hours; restless sleep 10.0%, 15.4%, 20.3%, and 30.3%; no nighttime awakenings 27.2%, 7.8%, 5.5%, and 1.9%. Sleep hygiene strategies are provided in Box 3.2. While benadryl is an FDA risk-category B drug that can be occasionally used during pregnancy, night time doses of benadryl plus acetaminophen combination products should be avoided, because daily or near daily use of analgesics may result in medication overuse headaches. Benadryl alone, however, is not associated with the development of medication overuse headache.

Box 3.2 Strategies for improving sleep

- Practice relaxation techniques at bedtime
- Use bed only for sleep and sex
  - Go to bed only when sleepy
  - Don't watch television or read in bed
- Establish and maintain regular sleep and rise times
- Avoid daytime naps if you have problems sleeping at night
- Reduce evening stimulants (caffeine, nicotine)
- Don't drink alcohol before going to bed
- Do aerobic exercise daily
- Make sure the temperature in the bedroom is comfortably cool
- If too much ambient light enters the bedroom, invest in an eye mask
- If noises in the bedroom prevent sleep, try using ear plugs
- If you are unable to fall asleep after 15 minutes, get up and go to another room. Only return to bed when you are sleepy.

Patients reporting snoring or sleep apnea may need to be evaluated for obstructive sleep apnea. A recent small study tested 35 pregnant women reporting snoring or apnea with polysomnography and nonstress test recordings during sleep [54]. Obstructive sleep apnea was diagnosed in four women (11%), with fetal heart decelerations recorded in conjunction with maternal desaturation in three of the four babies. Furthermore, birth weight and Apgar scores were lower in the newborns born to those women diagnosed with obstructive sleep apnea.

> *Pearl for the practitioner:*
> Pregnant women reporting snoring or sleep apnea may need to be evaluated for obstructive sleep apnea, which is associated with fetal distress.

Smoking

Consuming nicotine-containing products alters several important neurochemicals that influence headache activity, including endorphins [55], serotonin, norepinephrine, and dopamine [56]. The ability of nicotine to alter these chemicals explains changes in feelings of anxiety and difficulty with discontinuation in smokers. Neurochemical changes may also result in increases in headache.

Smokers are more likely to develop chronic headaches compared with nonsmokers. For example, current smokers are 35% more likely to develop migraines compared with people who have never smoked [57]. Furthermore, headache frequency and severity are increased in heavier nicotine users [58]. Smoking cessation has been reported anecdotally to reduce headache activity; however, no controlled studies have been conducted in migraineurs.

> *Pearl for the practitioner:*
> Smokers are more likely to develop chronic headaches than nonsmokers. Headache frequency and severity are also increased in heavier nicotine users. Smoking cessation likely may improve headaches, although controlled studies are lacking.

Smoking and pregnancy

Nicotine has been linked to increased headache activity during pregnancy. A longitudinal survey of 4,761 women experiencing a pregnancy over a 3.5 year period reported severe headache significantly more often in smokers compared with nonsmokers (22% vs. 17%, $P<0.001$) [59]. Smoking cessation is recommended during pregnancy for a variety of health reasons. Although headache reduction has not specifically been tested in pregnant headache sufferers, clinical experience suggests that headache improvement may occur with smoking cessation. Patients can learn about effective programs to facilitate nicotine discontinuation through local medical resources or national initiatives, such as 1-800-QUIT-NOW (1-800-784-8669), developed by the United States Department of Health and Human Services, National Institutes of Health, and National Cancer Institute. Smokers can receive a free smoking cessation plan and coach through the 1-800-QUIT-NOW phone number or the website: (http://1800quitnow.cancer.gov).

> **Pearl for the practitioner:**
> Smoking cessation is important for all smokers, especially those who are pregnant or breastfeeding. A plan to quit smoking and a coach to provide advice can be accessed by calling 1-800-QUIT-NOW.

Exercise and Physical Therapy

Musculoskeletal abnormalities are present in the majority of migraineurs, with postural abnormalities in 83% and myofascial trigger points in 79% [60]. Whether musculoskeletal changes represent a primary cause of head pain or a secondary consequence, therapy targeting muscles can help reduce contributory musculoskeletal dysfunction, as well as reduce pain by enhancing release of pain-relieving chemicals like endorphins. Aerobic exercise, targeted neck exercises, and oral appliances have demonstrated benefit for headache reduction. Specific headache-reducing exercise instruction is provided in Chapter 10 and on the accompanying CD.

Aerobic Exercise

Aerobic exercise showed benefit as headache prevention in a controlled study randomizing migraineurs to standard aerobic exercise 3 times per week for 6 weeks, or a wait list control [61]. Pain severity decreased by 44% and pain duration by 36% in the exercise group. There were no changes in headache activity in the control group. Although the reduction in headache activity did not reach clinical significance (50% reduction), the authors hypothesized that the lack of any improvement in the control group, as is typically seen, suggested that those improvements seen in the treated group were more significant than a placebo response.

Stretching Exercises

Stretching exercises of the neck may help reduce headache frequency, as well as acutely reduce pain during a headache episode. Performing stretching exercises in the shower or warm bath or first putting a heating pad on the neck for 15 minutes may achieve a more complete and effective stretch. If pain persists after stretching, ice packs may help. Postural correction, deep muscle massage, and other physical therapy modalities may also help reduce headache pain. Correcting imbalances between opposing muscle groups can further lessen muscle tension and tightness, which may lead to decreased pain.

A crossover treatment study comparing outcome between two non-drug treatments showed good relief from relaxation/biofeedback but not physical therapy as first-line treatment [62]. Initial treatment with physical therapy was beneficial for only 14%, compared with 41% treated with relaxation/biofeedback. When used as adjunctive therapy, 47% who failed to achieve benefit with relaxation/biofeedback alone did experience significant headache reduction when physical therapy was added. Physical therapy may, therefore, be a useful adjunctive treatment for those who failed an initial course of relaxation or biofeedback.

Intraoral Appliances

Contraction of craniomandibular muscles may contribute to headache activity. Effective methods to reduce muscle tension include relaxation techniques, exercise, and intraoral splints. Intraoral appliances have demonstrated efficacy in patients with primary headache, like migraine [63]. For example, in a small study of 19 migraineurs treated with nocturnal occlusal appliances, the number of migraine attacks was reduced by 40% [64].

The Nociceptive Trigeminal Inhibition (NTI) appliance is an FDA-approved migraine prevention treatment (www.nti-tss.com). This acrylic mini-splint fits over the incisors to reduce jaw clenching, which may contribute to increased headache activity. In a randomized study, migraine patients with pericranial muscle tenderness were treated with either a full coverage occlusal splint or the NTI mini-splint [65]. All patients wore splints for two months at night and during times of stress. After eight weeks, migraine frequency decreased by 38% in the full occlusal splint group, similar to results from the earlier small study referenced above [64]. Migraineurs randomized to the NTI splint experienced significantly greater improvement, with a 62% decrease in migraine frequency ($P<0.05$). Oral devices, therefore, may offer a safe and effective alternative for patients with headache and associated pericranial muscle tenderness during pregnancy and lactation.

Massage and Other Manual Therapies

Muscular tension and contraction in the head, neck, and shoulder girdle frequently accompany symptoms of headache. Massage of the temples, head, and neck is often perceived as soothing during a headache attack, particularly for tension-type headache. Although data are limited, a review of the literature suggests some modest benefit from massage therapy for migraine and tension-type headaches [66]. Therefore, while massage should not be used as monotherapy, it may provide adjunctive benefit, especially for more severe headache episodes, to reduce pain and permit performing stretching exercises. Treating muscle tension with therapeutic massage can result in decreased pain and stress, with minimal side effects, making this a particularly attractive option for women during pregnancy and breastfeeding. Acupuncture has been extensively evaluated for headache treatment; however, randomized studies consistently show no better results in patients treated with acupuncture compared with placebo [67].

Limited data are available to evaluate the benefit of other manual therapies, such as chiropractic care, spinal manipulation, and craniosacral therapy. A recent review of studies evaluating manual therapies in patients with tension-type headache concluded that available data from well-designed studies was insufficient to permit uniformly recommending these therapies [68]. Most studies have evaluated the benefits of spinal manipulation and mobilization. Although anecdotal reports of success have been reported, controlled data are limited [69,70]. Patients with pronounced musculoskeletal changes or consistent headache triggering by deviations in posture or exertion of neck muscles may be the best candidates for manual therapy.

Summary

A wide variety of effective and safe non-drug options are available for the pregnant and breastfeeding headache sufferer to use as monotherapy or in conjunction with medications. Beneficial non-drug headache treatments that can be useful during preconception, pregnancy, and lactation include pain management techniques (such as relaxation, biofeedback, and stress management); smoking cessation; and lifestyle regulation. Food elimination diets are generally not helpful for reducing headaches and are discouraged for pregnant and nursing mothers to avoid eliminating necessary nutrients. Headaches may be reduced by regularly eating meals and snacks and achieving adequate hydration. Select patients may benefit from additional treatment with aerobic exercise, physical therapy, and manual therapies.

Practical pointers:

- Offering instruction in non-drug treatments before conception allows the woman to develop effective non-pharmacological skills while she still has access to a full armamentarium of rescue medications.
- Non-pharmacological therapies are safe and effective and should be used as part of a comprehensive headache treatment regimen.
- The most effective non-drug treatments are stress management, relaxation, and lifestyle modifications. Aerobic exercise, physical therapy, and manual treatments can supplement other non-pharmacological skills.
- Non-drug treatments can be used as monotherapy for mild headaches and in conjunction with safer medications for more severe attacks.
- Patients should limit exposure to modifiable triggers like fasting, sleep deprivation, and nicotine. Excessive focus on trigger avoidance can be counterproductive.
- Patients should concentrate on using active non-drug treatments like relaxation, stress management, exercise, and regular scheduling of meals and sleep.

References

1. Bag B, Karabulut N. Pain-relieving factors in migraine and tension-type headache. *Int J Clin Pract* 2005;59:760–763.
2. Rothrock JF, Parada VA, Sims C, et al. The impact of intensive patient education on clinical outcome in a clinic-based migraine population. *Headache* 2006;46:726–731.
3. Holroyd KA, France JC, Cordingley GE. Enhancing the effectiveness of relaxation-thermal biofeedback training with propranolol hydrochloride. *J Consult Clin Psychol* 1995;63:327–330.
4. Scharff L, Turk DC, Marcus DA. Headache triggers and coping responses of different diagnostic groups. *Headache* 1995;35:397–403.
5. Kelman L. The triggers or precipitants of the acute migraine attack. *Cephalalgia* 2007;27:394–402.
6. Martin PR, Todd J, Reece J. Effects of noise and a stressor on head pain. *Headache* 2005;45:1353–1364.
7. Medina JC, Diamond S. The role of diet in migraine. *Headache* 1978;18:31–34.
8. Koehler SM, Glaros A. The effect of aspartame on migraine headache. *Headache* 1988;28:10–14.
9. Marcus DA, Scharff L, Turk DC, Gourley LM. A double-blind provocative study of chocolate as a trigger for headache. *Cephalalgia* 1997;17:855–862.
10. Kelman L. The premonitory symptoms (prodrome): a tertiary care study of 893 migraineurs. *Headache* 2004;44:865–872.
11. Martin PR. How do trigger factors acquire the capacity to precipitate headaches? *Behav Res Ther* 2001;39:545–554.
12. Martin PR, Reece J, Forsyth M. Noise as a trigger for headaches: relationship between exposure and sensitivity. *Headache* 2006;46:962–972.

13. Martin PR, Lae L, Reece J. Stress as a trigger for headaches: relationship between exposure and sensitivity. *Anxiety Stress Coping* 2007;20:393–407.
14. Mathew RC, Ho BT, Kralik P, Claghorn JL. Biochemical basis for biofeedback treatment of migraine: a hypothesis. *Headache* 1979;19:290–293.
15. Warner G, Lance JW. Relaxation therapy in migraine and chronic tension headache. *Med J Australia* 1975;1:298–301.
16. Daly EJ, Donn PA, Galliher MJ, Zimmerman JS. Biofeedback applications to migraine and tension headache: a double-blinded outcome study. *Biofeedback & Self-Regulation* 1983;8:135–152.
17. Kaushik R, Kaushik RM, Mahajan SK, Rajesh V. Biofeedback assisted diaphragmatic breathing and systematic relaxation versus propranolol in long term prophylaxis of migraine. *Complement Ther Med* 2005;13:165–174.
18. Marcus DA, Scharff L, Turk DC. Nonpharmacologial management of headaches during pregnancy. *Psychosom Med* 1995;57:527–535.
19. Scharff L, Marcus DA, Turk DC. Maintenance of effects in the nonmedical treatment of headaches during pregnancy. *Headache* 1996;36:285–290.
20. Mäki K, Vahtera J, Virtanen M, et al. Work stress and new-onset migraine in a female employee population. *Cephalalgia* 2008;28:18–25.
21. Chaouloff F, Berton O, Mormed P. Serotonin and stress. *Neuropsychopharmacology* 1999;21(Suppl 2):S28–S32.
22. Tomaszewska D, Mateusiak K, Przekop F. Changes in extracellular LHRH and beta-endorphin-like immunoreactivity in the nucleus infundibularis-median eminence of anestrous ewes under stress. *J Neural Transm* 1999;106:265–274.
23. Tomaszewska D, Przekop F. Catecholamine activity in the medial preoptic area and nucleus infundibularis-median eminence of anestrous ewes in normal physiological state and under stress. *J Neural Transm* 1999;106:1031–1043.
24. Fernandez E, Sheffield J. Relative contributions of life events versus daily hassles to the frequency and intensity of headache. *Headache* 1996;36:595–602.
25. Kohlenberg RT, Cahn T. Self-help treatment for migraine headaches: a controlled outcome study. *Headache* 1981;21:196–200.
26. Mitchell KR, White RG. Control of migraine headache by behavioral self-management: a controlled case study. *Headache* 1976;16:178–184.
27. Cordingley G, Holrody K, Pingel J, Jerome A, Nash J. Amitriptyline versus stress management therapy in the prophylaxis of chronic tension headache. *Headache* 1990;30:300.
28. French DJ, Holroyd KA, Pinell C, Malinoski PT, O'Donnell F, Hill KR. Perceived self-efficacy and headache-related disability. *Headache* 2000;40:647–656.
29. Mérelle SM, Sorbi MJ, van Doornen LP, Passchier J. Migraine patients as trainers of their fellow patients in non-pharmacological prevention attack management: short-term effects of a randomized controlled trial. *Cephalalgia* 2007;28:127–138.
30. Nicholson R, Nash J, Andrasik F. A self-administered behavioral intervention using tailored messages for migraine. *Headache* 2005;45:1124–1139.
31. Cottrell C, Drew J, Gibson J, Holroyd K, O'Donnell F. Feasibility assessment of telephone-administered behavioral treatment for adolescent migraine. *Headache* 2007;47:1293–1302.
32. Devineni T, Blanchard EB. A randomized controlled trial of an internet-based treatment for chronic headache. *Behav Res Ther* 2005;43:277–292.
33. Medina JL, Diamond S. The role of diet in migraine. *Headache* 1978;18:31–34.
34. Mosek A, Korczyn AD. Yom Kippur headache. *Neurology* 1995;45:1953–1955.
35. Topacoglu H, Karcioglu O, Yuruktumen A, et al. Impact of Ramadan on demographics and frequencies of disease-related visits in the emergency department. *Int J Clin Pract* 2005;59:900–905.
36. Montgomery KS. Nutrition column: an update on water needs during pregnancy and beyond. *J Perinat Educ* 2002;11:40–42.

37. Spigt MG, Kuijper EC, Schayck CP, et al. Increasing daily water intake for prophylactic treatment of headache: a pilot trial. *Eur J Neurol* 2005;12:715–718.
38. Goh YI, Bollano E, Einarson TR, Koren G. Prenatal multivitamin supplementation and rates of congenital anomalies: a meta-analysis. *J Obstet Gynaecol Can* 2006;28:680–689.
39. Centers for Disease Control. Folate status in women of childbearing age – United States, 1999. *MMWR* 2000;49:962–965.
40. Centers for Disease Control. Recommendations for the use of folic acid to reduce the number of cases of spina bifida and other neural tube defects. *MMWR* 1992;41:001.
41. Marcus DA. Chronic headache: the importance of trigger identification. *Headache & Pain* 2003;14:139–144.
42. Toglia JU. Melatonin: a significant contributor to the pathogenesis of migraine. *Med Hypoth* 2001;57:432–434.
43. Claustrat B, Loisy C, Brun J, et al. Nocturnal plasma melatonin levels in migraine: a preliminary report. *Headache* 1989;29:242–245.
44. Mauskop A, Altura BT, Altura BM. Serum ionized magnesium levels and serum ionized calcium/ionized magnesium ratios in women with menstrual migraine. *Headache* 2002;42:242–248.
45. Johnson S. The multifaceted and widespread pathology of magnesium deficiency. *Med Hypotheses* 2001;56:163–170.
46. Trauninger A, Pfund Z, Koszegi T, Czopf J. Oral magnesium load test in patients with migraine. *Headache* 2002;42:114–119.
47. Durlach J, Pages N, Bac P, Bara M, Guiet-Bara A. Biorhythms and possible central regulation of magnesium status, phototherapy, darkness therapy and chronopathological forms of magnesium depletion. *Magnes Res* 2002;15:49–66.
48. Chollet D, Franken P, Raffin Y, et al. Blood and brain magnesium in inbred mice and their correlation with sleep quality. *Am J Physiol Regulatory Integrative Comp Physiol* 2000;279:R2173–R2178.
49. Takase B, Akima T, Satomura K, et al. Effects of chronic sleep deprivation on autonomic activity by examining heart rate variability, plasma catecholamine, and intracellular magnesium levels. *Biomed Pharmacother* 2004;58(suppl 1):S35–S39.
50. Boardman HF, Thomas E, Millson DS, Croft PR. Psychological, sleep, lifestyle, and comorbid associations with headache. *Headache* 2005;45:657–669.
51. Gori S, Morelli N, Maestri M, et al. Sleep quality, chronotypes and preferential timing of attacks in migraine without aura. *J Headache Pain* 2005;6:258–260.
52. Kelman L, Rains JC. Headache and sleep: examination of sleep patterns and complaints in a large clinical sample of migraineurs. *Headache* 2005;45:904–910.
53. Hedman C, Pohjasvaara T, Tolonen U, Suhonen-Malm AS, Myllylä VV. Effects of pregnancy on mothers' sleep. *Sleep Med* 2002;3:37–42.
54. Salin FK, Koken G, Cosar E, et al. Obstructive sleep apnea in pregnancy and fetal outcome. *Int J Gynaecol Obstet* 2008;100:141–146.
55. Pomerleau OF. Endogenous opioids and smoking – a review of progress and problems. *Psychoneuroendocrinology* 1998;23:115–130.
56. Mansbach RS, Rovetti CC, Freeland CS. The role of monoamine neurotransmitters system in the nicotine discriminative stimulus. *Drug Alcohol Depend* 1998;23:115–130.
57. Hozawa A, Houston T, Steffes MW, et al. The association of cigarette smoking with self-reported disease before middle age: the Coronary Artery Risk Development in Young Adults (CARDIA) study. *Prev Med* 2006;42:193–199.
58. Payne TJ, Stetson B, Stevens VM, Johnson CA, Penzien DB, Van Dorsten B. Impact of cigarette smoking on headache activity in headache patients. *Headache* 1991;31:329–332.
59. Christian P, West KP, Katz J, et al. Cigarette smoking during pregnancy in rural Nepal. Risk factors and effects of beta-carotene and vitamin A supplementation. *Eur J Clin Nutr* 2004;58:204–211.

60. Marcus DA, Scharff L, Mercer SR, Turk DC. Musculoskeletal abnormalities in chronic headache: a controlled comparison of headache diagnostic groups. *Headache* 1999;39:21–27.
61. Lockett DC, Campbell JF. The effects of aerobic exercise on migraine. *Headache* 1992;32:50–54.
62. Marcus DA, Scharff L, Mercer SR, Turk DC. Nonpharmacological treatment for migraine: incremental utility of physical therapy with relaxation and thermal biofeedback. *Cephalalgia* 1998;18:266–272.
63. Shevel E. Craniomandibular muscles, intraoral orthoses and migraine. *Expert Rev Neurotherapeutics* 2005;5:371–377.
64. Lamey PJ, Steele JG, Aitchison T. Migraine: the effect of acrylic appliance design on clinical response. *Br Dent J* 1996;180:137–140.
65. Shankland WE. Migraine and tension-type headache reduction through pericranial muscular suppression: a preliminary report. *Cranio* 2001;19:269–278.
66. Tsao JI. Effectiveness of massage therapy for chronic, non-malignant pain: a review. *Evid Based Complement Alternat Med* 2007;4:165–179.
67. Schürks M, Diener H, Goadsby P. Update on the prophylaxis of migraine. *Curr Treat Opt Neurol* 2008;10:20–29.
68. Fernández-de-Las-Peñas C, Alonso-Blanco C, Cuardrado ML, et al. Are manual therapies effective in reducing pain from tension-type headache? a systematic review. *Clin J Pain* 2006;22:278–285.
69. Astin JA, Ernst E. The effectiveness of spinal manipulation for the treatment of headache disorders: a systematic review of randomized clinical trials. *Cephalalgia* 2002;22:617–623.
70. Fernández-de-Las-Peñas C, Alonso-Blanco C, San-Roman J, Miangolarra-Page JC. Methodological quality of randomized controlled trials of spinal manipulation and mobilization in tension-type headache, migraine, and cervicogenic headache. *J Orthop Sports Phys Ther* 2006;36:160–169.

Chapter 4
Acute Treatment Options for the Pregnant Headache Patient

Key Chapter Points

- Many pregnant women will take prescription and non-prescription medications to treat their acute headaches with or without their practitioner's knowledge.
- Regular use of acute medications should be limited to two days per week or less to prevent medication overuse (rebound) headaches from developing. Patients with more frequent headaches should consider preventive therapy.
- Safer treatment strategies need to be explicitly outlined during preconception planning and reviewed at each office visit during the pregnancy.
- Acute prescription headache medications during pregnancy are generally limited to acetaminophen, intranasal lidocaine, rescue opioids, and anti-emetics.
- Effective non-drug acute migraine treatments include relaxation, biofeedback, distraction, exercise, and acupressure. Topical peppermint oil may also be used.
- A variety of prescription medications, supplements, and non-drug therapies may be used adjunctively to reduce migraine-related nausea during pregnancy.
- General principles for treating acute headaches in pregnant women include not treating mild headaches, treating nausea aggressively, maximizing non-drug options, and, if medications are to be used, using the safest medications for the shortest time at the lowest dose as late in the pregnancy as possible.

Keywords Acute migraine · Herbal · Nausea · Vitamin

When Sarah attended her first obstetrical appointment, she excitedly informed her practitioner, "I'm thrilled to finally be having a baby! I really want this pregnancy to be perfect and I'm not going to use any medications besides my vitamins and iron!" Satisfied that she was planning to utilize previously taught non-medication techniques for her migraines, specific medication recommendations were not given. When Sarah returned the following month for her second visit, she reported using a prescription for hydrocodone plus ibuprofen (Vicoprofen) once weekly for bad headaches, using leftover pills that had been previously prescribed for a dental procedure. She was also using daily over-the-counter antacids and naproxen (Aleve) 3 times weekly. She used licorice one week when

D.A. Marcus, P.A. Bain, *Effective Migraine Treatment in Pregnant and Lactating Women: A Practical Guide*, DOI 10.1007/978-1-60327-439-5_4,
© Humana Press, a part of Springer Science+Business Media, LLC 2009

*she had a bad cough, and was starting to take ginger supplements to combat morning
sickness and headaches.*

Clinicians are often apprehensive about treating headaches in pregnant women.
Ideally, medication therapy would be limited to infrequent use during later
pregnancy to minimize medication-related risks for the developing baby.
Migraines, however, are often disabling, especially during the first trimester,
and untreated severe episodes can lead to nausea, vomiting, and dehydration,
which can be detrimental to the fetus. Practitioners often warn against using
any medications during pregnancy, but patients may panic during an acute
attack and take whatever they have available. Despite efforts to minimize
medications during pregnancy, however, many migraineurs use acute therapies—with or without their practitioner's knowledge and approval, as seen in
the case above. A frank, open discussion with the patient about appropriate use
of safer medications before conception or during early pregnancy is essential to
achieve optimal headache care.

> **Pearl for the practitioner:**
> Many migraine sufferers take medications to treat their headaches and
> nausea—with or without the knowledge and advice of their practitioner.
> A relatively safe, effective treatment plan needs to be explicitly developed
> with the patient, ideally prior to conception, and reviewed throughout
> pregnancy.

Typical medication use during pregnancy has been studied in several
epidemiological surveys. An observational study of 418 pregnant women
found that, after excluding prenatal vitamins and iron, three in four
women used at least one additional prescription and nearly two in three
used over-the-counter (OTC) drugs during their pregnancies (Fig. 4.1) [1].
The most frequently used prescription, OTC, and herbal remedies included
analgesics and treatments to combat nausea, both of which might be used
for acute migraine treatment (Table 4.1). Data about medication use during
pregnancy from two large national surveys of ambulatory patients in the
United States similarly showed that, after vitamins and iron, antibiotics,
hypoglycemics, and analgesics were the next most commonly prescribed
medications during pregnancy [2]. Review of medication usage in Australia
found surprisingly comparable results, with pregnant women using an average of one prescribed and two non-prescribed medications during pregnancy, with analgesics, vitamins, and antacids the most commonly used
drug categories (Fig. 4.2) [3]. Interestingly, this study highlights that, while
pregnant women like Sarah often express a desire to reduce medication
usage during pregnancy, analgesic consumption is not substantially less for
most gravid women compared with their pre-pregnancy use.

Pearl for the practitioner:
While most pregnant women want to minimize medication use during pregnancy, a substantial number will take prescription and non-prescription medications.

Statistics regarding safe medication use in pregnant women are not as robust as in non-pregnant women, due to lack of adequate controlled clinical trial data in pregnant patients. Sufficient data, however, are available to aid

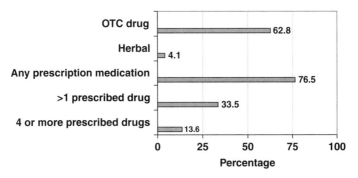

Fig. 4.1 Medication use during pregnancy (Based on [1])
Medication use excludes use of prenatal vitamins and iron. OTC=over-the-counter.

Table 4.1 Top medications used during pregnancy (Based on [1])

Medication type	Specific drug	Percentage of women using
Prescription	Metronidazole	9.1
	Acetaminophen with codeine	8.4
	Cephalexin	7.4
	Albuterol	7.0
	Terconazole	5.8
	Azithromycin	4.1
Over-the-counter	Acetaminophen	39.6
	Antacids	25.9
	Ibuprofen	10.1
	Cough syrup	6.5
	Aspirin	4.8
Herbal	Garlic	1.0
	Ginseng	1.0
	Melatonin	0.5
	Ginkgo	0.5
	Licorice	0.5
	Ginger	0.2
	Cod liver oil	0.2

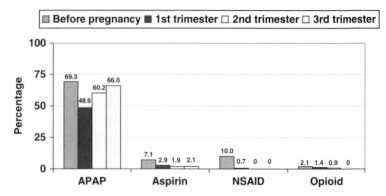

Fig. 4.2 Medication usage before and during pregnancy (Based on [3])
Data were collected to compare medication usage during the three months before conception and each trimester. Medication usage during pregnancy was confirmed by reviewing medical records. APAP = paracetamol/acetaminophen. NSAID = non-steroidal anti-inflammatory drug. The only significant differences in analgesic usage after pregnancy were a significant reduction of acetaminophen usage during the first trimester ($P<0.01$) and NSAIDs during each trimester ($P<0.05$).

the clinician in making safer, reasonable treatment recommendations. Clinicians should be aware that, without appropriate direction about migraine treatment during pregnancy, many pregnant women will self-medicate. Healthcare providers need to develop effective approaches for the treatment of acute migraine that will include recommendations for both non-medication and medication therapies, even when medication will be reserved as rescue treatment only. Failure to effectively develop approved medication recommendations with patients will likely lead to unnecessary suffering and/or self-medication by the patient.

Design Safer Treatment Plans Before Conception

Every woman of reproductive potential should be educated about likely headache changes with pregnancy, as well as the need to adjust therapies to ensure the best fetal outcome. Information about lifestyle management, as well as pain management skill training, is appropriate for all female patients in preparation for possible conception. Women with migraine should have available relatively safe, acute therapies when severe attacks occur to avoid unnecessary disability and dehydration.

Treating clinicians should approach each female in her reproductive years with preconception counseling to inform women about expected changes in headache patterns during pregnancy and safer treatment options. Sexually active patients who do not consistently use effective contraception should be treated with therapies that may be safely used during early pregnancy to avoid possible early teratogenic effects when women may not initially realize they are

Box 4.1 Guidelines for treating migraine in fertile women

- Ask about current method of contraception
- Ask about plans for conception
- Describe necessary changes to current treatment regimen before planned conception
- Revise treatment plan to include medications permissible during pregnancy if:

    - Patient does not consistently use effective contraception
    - Patient is ready to attempt conception
    - Patient identifies she is or might be pregnant

pregnant (Box 4.1). Patients should understand that, while the majority of women experience migraine improvement during pregnancy, migraine may worsen (especially during the first trimester) or continue unchanged. In addition, postpartum migraine treatment plans should be made well in advance of delivery. Discussing headache treatment proactively often opens important doors of communication to patient concerns about general health, reproductive issues, and headache changes over a woman's lifetime.

Pearl for the practitioner:
Proactively discussing a treatment plan for headaches during pregnancy with all women of reproductive potential is important.

Develop a Safer and Effective Acute Treatment Plan

The most serious medication effects on the fetus occur with early exposure, before many women are aware that they are pregnant. Therefore, management of young women with chronic headache needs to include an evaluation of reproductive status and contraceptive use. Women planning for pregnancy, as well as fertile women not using effective contraception and at risk for pregnancy, should be treated with those medications deemed relatively safe during early pregnancy. Four main principles guide acute migraine treatment in pregnant headache sufferers:

- Don't medicate mild headaches.
- Treat nausea aggressively and avoid dehydration.
- Maximize non-drug approaches.

- Use medications safely:

  - The lowest dose;
  - The safest medications;
  - For the shortest time;
  - As late in the pregnancy as possible.

Don't Medicate Mild Headaches

Non-pregnant women are often instructed to medicate their headaches early during mild symptom severity stages to maximize success. While this approach is effective, it can also lead to treating headache attacks that might have responded to non-drug monotherapy. In the pregnant patient, minimizing medications becomes a higher priority, so this group should be instructed to not treat milder headaches with medication but to use non-drug options first. Patients should be encouraged to utilize a step approach to migraine treatment during pregnancy (Fig. 4.3). For example, a woman may report that if she treats her migraine when the severity is still mild, relaxation and distraction alone are effective. When she recognizes a moderate severity headache early, she may need to add heat or ice, stretching, and/or acupressure. When pain is severe at onset, medication therapy may be needed right away to prevent the pain from becoming incapacitating or reduce the chance that symptoms will progress to include overt vomiting. Most women are encouraged to have an armamentarium of treatment options available in order to have a rational step-wise plan of care.

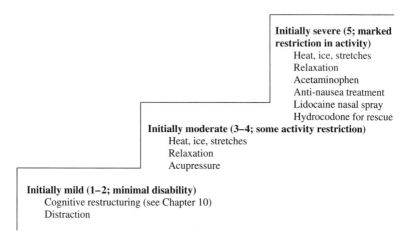

Fig. 4.3 Sample step acute migraine care, based on symptom severity
Pain scale based on 0–5 scale with 0 = no headache and 5 = disabling headache. Severity should be linked with disability more than pain severity. *Mild headache* is associated with no or minimal activity restriction. *Moderate headache* is associated with some restriction of activity. *Severe headache* should be associated with substantial disability.

Because patients interpret pain severity levels differently and have different tolerances to various levels of discomfort, it is more useful to encourage patients to rate headache severity based on level of functional disability rather than pain levels. Using this system, *mild headache* is associated with no or minimal activity restriction. *Moderate headache* is associated with some restriction of activity. *Severe headache* should be associated with substantial disability. Patients able to continue to function with their headache will often achieve success with non-drug treatments. Even though patients may report a migraine pain severity of 8 or 9 on a 0–10 severity scale (0 = no pain, 10 = excruciating pain), if there are no impairments in functional ability, that headache should be rated as *mild*. Patients thus learn that medications are designed to reduce disability rather than simply relieve migraine discomfort, which can often be achieved through non-drug treatments.

> **Pearl for the practitioner:**
> Ask patients to rate headache disability rather than headache pain severity when deciding which treatments to recommend.

Treat Nausea Aggressively

Nausea is most common during the first trimester and can be quite severe at times. Unfortunately, migraine is also most likely to be more frequent and severe during the first trimester, and migraine may increase nausea complaints. Furthermore, dehydration can be a potent trigger for headaches. Nausea should be minimized to reduce disability, maximize good nutrition, and prevent dehydration. Suboptimal maternal nutrition in early pregnancy may affect fetal growth and development [4]. Although most studies evaluating the effects of nutritional deficits or dehydration during pregnancy are related to nausea and vomiting from hyperemesis gravidarum, severe and frequent migraine may also contribute to dehydration and periods of poor nutrition. Preventing dehydration and ensuring good nutrition are important considerations for using anti-emetic medications during pregnancy. There are safer, effective medications available to treat nausea during pregnancy.

> **Pearl for the practitioner:**
> Treat pregnancy-related nausea aggressively to avoid dehydration and disability.

Non-drug Treatments

Dietary adjustments can help reduce pregnancy-related nausea. (A patient handout regarding dietary suggestions for women with persistent nausea is available in Chapter 10 and on the accompanying CD.) Nauseated patients should avoid exposure to strong odors and drink bland liquids. Diluting carbonated beverages and juices 1:1 with water may improve fluid intake. Nausea may also be curbed by snacking on easily digested, bland foods, such as crackers, applesauce, bananas, rice, and pasta.

Acupressure over the wrist can also relieve nausea. Patients can stimulate acupressure point P6 by applying gentle, massaging pressure on the volar aspect (palm side) of the wrist, two fingerbreadths proximal to the wrist crease. (Acupressure instructions for patients are similarly provided in Chapter 10 and the accompanying CD.) OTC Sea-Band^{TM} wristbands can also activate this acupressure point and reduce nausea.

> *Pearl for the practitioner:*
> Dietary suggestions and acupressure point stimulation can help reduce mild to moderate nausea during pregnancy.

Anti-emetic Medications

There are a number of safer, effective medication options to treat nausea, using several routes of administration, including rectal, orally disintegrating, and topical preparations (Table 4.2). A recent survey of practicing obstetricians identified promethazine and ondansetron as the most commonly prescribed anti-emetics during pregnancy [5]. Metoclopramide and ondansetron are rated FDA risk-category B and are considered safe for use in pregnancy. Promethazine is FDA risk-category C.

> *Pearl for the practitioner:*
> Metoclopramide and ondansetron are rated FDA risk-category B and are considered safe for use in pregnancy to treat nausea. Promethazine is rated FDA risk-category C, but is commonly used by obstetricians.

Herbs and Supplements

Recommendations from the American College of Obstetricians and Gynecologists include utilization of herbal and vitamin supplements for nausea, including vitamin B6 and ginger [6]. A recent review of six randomized, double-blind clinical trials showed that ginger was as effective as B6 and more effective than placebo for relieving pregnancy-related nausea and vomiting, with safety supported by observational data [7]. Data from two representative randomized comparative studies are shown in Fig. 4.4 [8,9]. While these data do not

Table 4.2 Recommended anti-nausea medications during pregnancy. All drugs are dosed as needed

Drug	FDA Class	Dose	Comments
Meclizine (Antivert, Bonine, Dramamine, Medivert)	B	12.5 mg–25 mg PO QD Chewable available	Sedation, OTC Mostly used for motion sickness, but safe and can help with nausea
Metoclopromide (Reglan)	B	5–10 mg PO QID Liquid available	Sedation, agitation
Phosphorated Carbohydrate Solution (Emetrol)	B	15–30 mL Q 15 minutes—max 5 doses/ day	OTC Safe Modest efficacy
Ondansetron (Emeset, Emetron, Ondemet, Zofran)	B	4–8 mg PO BID Liquid and ODT available	Safe Well tolerated Preferred by obstetricians
Doxylamine	B	25 mg PO QID	In USA, marketed as sleep aid, Unisom Preferred nausea agent outside of USA
Promethazine (Phenergen, Promethegan)	C	12.5–25 mg PO/PR QID Injection available	Preferred by obstetricians Sedation, restlessness Narrow angle glaucoma contraindicated
Prochlorperazine (Compazine)	C	5–10 mg PO TID-QID or 25 mg PR BID or 0.5 ml of 50 mg/mL topical gel applied to wrists every 4–6 hours	Sedation, agitation, ECG abnormalities
Chlorpromazine (Thorazine)	C	10–25 mg PO/PR QID Suppository not readily available	Restlessness, sedation
Hydroxyzine (Vistaril)	C	25–50 mg PO QID Liquid available	Sedation

ODT = orally disintegrating tablet, OTC = over-the-counter drug, PO = by mouth, PR = rectal, Q = every, QD = daily, QID = four times daily, TID = three times daily.

All drugs should be used as needed. Recommendations are based on clinical experience and FDA risk category, due to paucity of adequate or controlled clinical trial data during pregnancy. Extensive clinical experience in pregnancy is available for metoclopramide, meclizine, prochlorperazine, promethazine, and chlorpromazine. Topical gel preparations may also be compounded for promethazine (12.5 mg/mL) and ondansetron (8 mg/mL).

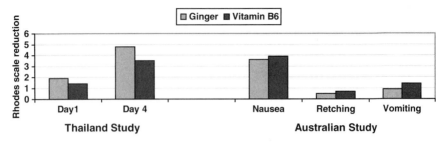

Fig. 4.4 Herbal and vitamin treatment of nausea during pregnancy (Based on [8,9])
In both studies, symptoms were rated using Rhodes scales, with possible scores ranging from 0 (no symptoms) to 12 (severe symptoms). In the Thailand study ($N = 123$), patients were treated with 650 mg ginger or 25 mg vitamin B6 three times daily for four days. Severity and duration of nausea/vomiting decreased progressively and significantly compared with baseline on each treatment day ($P<0.01$), with days 1 and 4 shown in the graph. Reductions on each day using ginger versus vitamin B6 (21.8% vs. 16.7% day 1 and 55.2% vs. 31.3% day 4) were significantly higher with ginger ($P<0.05$). In the Australian study ($N = 291$), patients were treated with 1.05 g ginger or 75 mg vitamin B6 once daily for 3 weeks. Reductions in symptoms occurred after 7 days and persisted for 3 weeks, with no significant differences between therapies. Individual symptom scales are shown for this study.

specifically target migraine-related nausea during pregnancy, ginger or vitamin B6 might additionally be useful treatments for nausea related to headache.

An-Tai-Yin is another herbal remedy sometimes used to treat morning sickness. An evaluation of outcome in 14,551 live births showed a link between the herbal treatment An-Tai-Yin (used during the first trimester by 11.4% of women) and congenital malformations [10]. Risk for musculoskeletal and connective tissue (odds ratio = 1.6) and eye malformations (odds ratio = 7.3) were significantly increased among offspring of women using An-Tai-Yin during the first trimester of pregnancy. Therefore, this treatment is not recommended.

Pearl for the practitioner:
Ginger and vitamin B6 are safe and effective supplement treatments for pregnancy-related nausea. Both are recommended by American College of Obstetricians and Gynecologists.

Determining First-Line Treatment of Migraine-Related Nausea During Pregnancy

The most commonly recommended treatments by practicing obstetricians for pregnancy-related nausea include supplements and behavioral therapy (Fig. 4.5) [5]. While supplements and behavioral therapy can be effective for mild nausea, moderate to severe nausea and/or vomiting should be aggressively

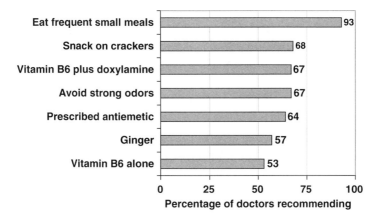

Fig. 4.5 Common obstetrician recommendations for nausea management (Based on [5])

treated with medications, such as metoclopromide, ondansetron, prochlorperazine, or promethazine. Figure 4.6 provides a recommended nausea treatment algorithm.

Combining anti-nausea therapies that act via different mechanisms may be more effective than using monotherapy. In a prospective, randomized study, combination treatment with pyridoxine (vitamin B6) plus metoclopromide was compared with monotherapy with either prochlorperazine or promethazine in 169 pregnant women during their first trimester [11]. Pyridoxine was administered as a 50 mg intramuscular injection with metoclopramide given 10 mg orally every 6 hours as needed. Prochlorperazine was administered as 25 mg rectal suppositories every 12 hours or 10 mg tablets every 6 hours as needed.

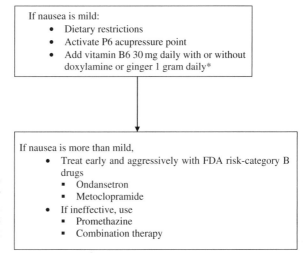

Fig. 4.6 Recommendations for treatment of nausea during conception and pregnancy
*Most studies have evaluated safety when using either supplement for 3–4 days. One study treated patients daily for 3 weeks, with good safety [9].

Promethazine was administered as 25 mg orally every 6 hours as needed. After treatment, emesis was reduced significantly more ($P<0.05$) with a pyridoxine-metoclopramide combination (74%) compared with prochlorperazine (52%) or promethazine (67%). Anecdotally, combining anti-nausea medications with different mechanisms of action, such as metoclopramide and ondansteron, can be particularly useful during an episode of severe nausea.

> **Pearl for the practitioner:**
> For particularly severe episodes of nausea, combining anti-emetics that work differently, such as metoclopramide and ondansetron, can be useful.

Maximize Non-drug Treatments

Healthy lifestyle changes (e.g., eating regular meals and not skipping meals, achieving adequate sleep, avoiding nicotine, and practicing stress management), physical therapy and exercise, and psychological pain management skills (e.g., relaxation, biofeedback, and stress management) are effective strategies to help minimize chronic primary headaches, like migraine and tension-type headaches (see Chapter 3). In general, most non-drug treatments work best as headache prevention, reducing headache frequency and severity. As described in Chapter 3, several non-drug treatments, such as relaxation, biofeedback, and stress management, can offer efficacy for migraine prevention similar to that of standard migraine prevention medications, when used in motivated patients [12]. Achieving acute headache relief with non-drug treatments alone is more difficult, achieving better success when techniques are used early, while headache severity is still mild to moderate, or when used in combination. Effective acute non-drug treatments include:

- Relaxation and biofeedback;
- Cognitive restructuring;
- Distraction;
- Oscillatory movements;
- Heat, ice, and neck stretches;
- Acupressure;
- Sleep regulation.

Specific details describing these techniques are provided in the Headache Treatment section of Chapter 10 and on the accompanying CD. Women should be encouraged to combine several techniques, such as applying a heating pad to the neck, using relaxation techniques, and performing neck stretches. By combining different modalities, patients can experience a greater impact on headache reduction.

> ***Pearl for the practitioner:***
> Benefit from non-drug treatments for acute headache reduction is max-
> imized by using techniques early when symptoms are still mild and com-
> bining different modalities.

Treat Co-existing Temporomandibular Dysfunction

During an acute headache attack, many headache patients experience tightening of their jaw muscles. Relieving this muscle tension acutely can help to
reduce headache pain. Furthermore, patients with co-existing temporomandibular dysfunction (TMD) may benefit from the addition of a nighttime
intraoral appliance or splint. TMD pain originates from the temporomandibular joint and surrounding muscles. Pain may be experienced in the jaw, face,
head, and neck. TMD pain typically improves with resting the jaw and
worsens with jaw opening. The normal jaw should open >40 mm (about
2 male knuckles wide) with no left or right deviation. Patients with TMD
characteristically show restricted opening, with jaw deviation, audible clicks
or popping, and discomfort. Isolated symptoms and signs of TMD occur in
half of all healthy adults without clinical TMD, especially masticatory muscle
tenderness in 12%, jaw deviation in 19%, and joint sounds in 25% [13].
Examination of 98 headache patients identified symptoms suggesting temporomandibular dysfunction in 55 patients (56%), with patients with the combination of both migraine and tension-type headaches most commonly affected
[14]. Accurate diagnosis of TMD must include identification of symptoms and
abnormalities with jaw movement. Benefits from intraoral devices alone are
typically short-lived, with long-term benefits superior when combining an
intraoral appliance with biofeedback and stress management [15]. Reducing
jaw muscle tightness, even in the absence of documented clinical TMD, can
help in an acute attack.

Effectively Implementing Non-drug Treatments

Just as women cannot learn Lamaze and other pain management strategies to
minimize labor discomfort after contractions have started, non-drug pain-
relieving therapies should be practiced between migraine episodes during the
training period. Ideally, non-drug skill training should begin during preconception before rescue medication options are limited. Women should also be
encouraged to proactively identify strategies for employing other non-drug
treatments, such as arranging for flexible break time at work, maintaining a
box of independent, quiet play activities to entertain young children for 20–30
minutes at home, and/or arranging for a friend or relative to help with

childcare during severe acute attacks. Having well-established contingency plans in place reduces the stress associated with disabling attacks that may occur at a time of increased responsibilities.

Select the Safest Effective Medications

Headache medications are divided into acute and preventive therapies. Acute therapies symptomatically treat individual headache episodes, while preventive therapies aim to reduce headache frequency. Regular use of all acute care medications needs to be limited to ≤2 days per week to avoid the development of medication overuse headache. Therefore, patients with migraine or tension-type headaches typically occurring >2 days per week should be treated with non-medication treatments and/or medication preventive therapies.

> *Pearl for the practitioner:*
> Regular use of all acute care medications needs to be limited to ≤2 days per week to avoid the development of medication overuse (rebound) headache.

Medication therapy during pregnancy is limited to minimize negative effects on the developing fetus. Updated information about medication effects during pregnancy can be obtained through pharmacists and Internet resources such as www.reprotox.org, www.motherisk.com, and others. As described in Chapter 2, medication safety during pregnancy may be categorized using the Food and Drug Administration (FDA) risk categories, with categories A-C available for treatment in women requiring medication treatments (Table 4.3). Women attempting conception or who are sexually active without reliable contraception should follow these same recommendations. While relatively safe, effective drugs are available to treat severe headaches in pregnant women, the number of available medication options is substantially restricted during pregnancy.

> *Pearl for the practitioner:*
> Women attempting conception or who are sexually active without reliable contraception should be treated with medications deemed safe during early pregnancy.

Patients with more severe migraines may fail to achieve adequate headache relief from non-medication therapy. In that case, consideration should be given to adding safer medications. Acute medications are designed to supplement rather than replace non-drug pain-relieving techniques.

Table 4.3 FDA risk classification of acute headache medications during attempted conception and pregnancy

	Relatively Safe (FDA risk category A or B)	Use if Benefit > Risk (FDA risk category C)	Avoid (FDA risk category D or X)
Acute medication	Acetaminophen [Tylenol] Caffeine Intranasal lidocaine NSAIDs 2nd trimester Ondansetron [Zofran] Prednisone	Low-dose aspirin Butalbital combination [Fiorinol, Fioricet][†] Dexamethasone NSAIDs 1st trimester[††] Opioids Prochlorperazine [Compazine] Promethazine [Phenergen, Promethegan] Triptans	Aspirin (other than low dose) Ergotamine [Cafergot, Wigraine] Isometheptene combination [Midrin] NSAIDs 3rd trimester

NSAID = non-steroidal anti-inflammatory drug

[†]Butalbital combination products are generally not recommended due to habit-forming properties and limited effectiveness in treating headache symptoms.

[††]While NSAIDs are technically FDA risk category B during the first two trimesters, data showing increased risk of miscarriage when used in early pregnancy suggest greater caution is necessary during the first trimester.

OTC Medications

OTC analgesics are commonly used by patients self-medicating for migraine. A survey of over 8,000 migraineurs in England and the United States showed that 52% of migraineurs used only OTC medications to treat their headaches [16]. Another 23% of migraineurs used both OTC and prescription medications. In both countries, the most commonly used OTC medication was acetaminophen, followed by ibuprofen (Motrin), and then caffeine/aspirin/acetaminophen combination products (like Excedrin). Unfortunately, this survey also showed that 75% of migraineurs in both countries still had substantial disability with their migraines, suggesting suboptimal relief from their treatments.

Although acetaminophen is generally less effective for acute headache than aspirin or non-steroidal anti-inflammatory drugs (NSAIDs), its safety is superior during pregnancy, due to a lack of significant effects by acetaminophen on the ductus arteriosus, uterine contractions, or bleeding. Furthermore, large epidemiological studies show no long-term effects in exposed babies [17].

> ***Pearl for the practitioner:***
> Acetaminophen is very safe during pregnancy and should be considered first-line acute medication treatment. Acetaminophen is available in a variety of forms, including tablets, capsules, suppositories, and liquids.

Early NSAID exposure has been linked to increased risk for miscarriage. A post hoc analysis of retrospectively collected data reported an 80% increased risk of miscarriage among NSAID users, with risk highest when NSAIDs were used around the time of conception [18]. In this same report, paracetamol (acetaminophen) use was not linked to increased miscarriage risk. While NSAIDs are generally restricted only during the third trimester in the United States, their use is limited to the second trimester in many European countries. Recent recommendations from the European Federation of Neurological Societies advised use of acetaminophen/paracetamol throughout pregnancy, with NSAIDs restricted to the second trimester [19]. While aspirin usage is restricted during pregnancy, women who have inadvertently used aspirin in early pregnancy can be comforted by data from a meta-analysis of the literature and a large epidemiological study using national registry data in Hungary, both of which showed no increased risk of congenital malformations among offspring of women using aspirin during the first trimester [20,21]. Furthermore, a large epidemiological study of 19,226 pregnancies showed no negative long-term effects on intellectual development in four-year-olds who had been exposed to aspirin during the first 20 weeks of gestation [22].

Pearl for the practitioner:
NSAIDs, if used, should be reserved for use in the second trimester only.

Caffeine can be a useful adjunctive therapy to enhance the pain-killing effect of analgesic medications and is rated FDA risk category B. In one study, adding 100 mg of caffeine to an analgesic increased the number of people experiencing migraine relief by 1.5 times [23]. While caffeine is often included in OTC analgesics, most also contain aspirin (e.g., Excedrin and Anacin), which is generally prohibited during pregnancy. Products combining only acetaminophen and caffeine (e.g., Excedrin Quick Tabs) are preferred during pregnancy. Alternatively, patients can supplement simple analgesic treatment (e.g., acetaminophen) with a caffeine-containing beverage. Typical amounts of caffeine in common beverages are:

- Coffee – 7 ounces – 65–135 mg caffeine;
- Espresso – 2 ounces – 100 mg caffeine;
- Tea – 7 ounces – 40–60 mg caffeine;
- Hot cocoa – 8 ounces – 14 mg caffeine;
- Cola – 12 ounces – 30–50 mg caffeine;
- Mountain Dew[TM] – 12 ounces – 54 mg caffeine;
- Red Bull[TM] – 8.2 ounces – 80 mg caffeine.

While consuming large amounts of caffeinated products would have undesirable stimulant effects, a recent literature review identified no clear increased malformation risk associated with maternal caffeine exposure [24]. Another large epidemiological study evaluated maternal caffeine consumption in 4,196 infants with cardiovascular malformations and 3,957 healthy infants, controlling for exposure to nicotine, alcohol, vasoactive medications, and folic acid supplementation [25]. No significant positive associations were identified between maternal caffeine consumption and cardiovascular malformation risk in exposed babies.

> **Pearl for the practitioner:**
> The analgesic effect of acetaminophen can be enhanced by adding moderate amounts of caffeine, which is rated FDA risk category B.

Prescription Medications

There are no adequate or well controlled studies in pregnant women for most prescription pain medications. In general, acetaminophen is recommended for the treatment of mild to moderate pain. For more severe pain, medications with the most clinical experience, such as hydrocodone (Vicodin) and morphine (MSIR, Roxanol), should be considered before others (Table 4.4).

Lidocaine is a FDA-B compound and is considered safe during pregnancy. Lidocaine may be compounded into a 4% nasal solution for intranasal use to treat headache. In a double-blind, randomized study, intranasal lidocaine provided short-lived (1–2 hours) of migraine relief for about half of treated, non-pregnant patients [26]. Patients should be instructed to lie down, extend the head over the edge of the bed and slowly drip 0.5–1 mL of 4% lidocaine (10–20 drops) into the nostril on the side of the headache, repeating 2 minutes later if needed. Although not specifically tested during pregnancy, intranasal lidocaine may help reduce reliance on opioid medications for treatment of more severe episodes.

Triptans are the most effective acute migraine agents, with their safety during pregnancy evaluated primarily in patient databases and voluntary registries [27]. The most extensive data are available for sumatriptan. In general, no high-quality evidence suggests an increased risk for malformations with maternal exposure to triptans. A Swedish database ($N = 658$ sumatriptan users) reported small, but not statistically significant, increased risks for preterm and low birth weight babies when mothers used sumatriptan [28]. Data, however, did not permit analysis of confounding factors, such as disease severity in sumatriptan users, which might have also influenced outcome. A recent review of available data on sumatriptan treatment concluded that first trimester treatment of worsening or new onset migraine is probably safe [29]. Due to the relatively small number of identified women who have used triptans during pregnancy, however, strong safety recommendations cannot be confidently made and triptans should generally be avoided during pregnancy. Clinicians are encouraged to report pregnancy outcomes of women exposed to triptans through company-sponsored registries. A complete list of available registries for medication exposures during pregnancy can

Table 4.4 Pain medication recommendations during pregnancy. All drugs are dosed as needed

Drug	FDA Class	Dose	Comments
Acetaminophen (Tylenol)	B	325–650 mg PO QID Liquid & PR available	Safe, inexpensive Not to exceed 4 g/day
Intranasal lidocaine	B	4% compounded solution. 0.5–1 mL. May repeat once.	Best studied for cluster headache. May help about half with migraine.
Hydrocodone (Vicodin, Lorcet, Lortab, Anexsia, Norco)	C	5–10 mg PO QID	Usually combined with APAP. Habit forming. Limit use near delivery due to fetal respiratory depression.
Non-steroidal anti-inflammatory drugs	C	Ibuprofen [Motrin] 400 mg PO TID-QID Liquid available Naproxen [Naprosyn] 500 mg PO, then 250 mg QID	Extensive use in pregnancy is reassuring. Limit use to 2nd trimester due to risk of miscarriage with early 1st trimester use.
Morphine (Astramorph, Duramorph, Infumorph, MSIR, Roxanol)	C	10–30 mg PO/SL TID-QID Liquid and injectable available	Itching, sedation Habit forming. Limit use near delivery due to fetal respiratory depression.
Oxycodone (Percocet)	B C (Australia)	5–30 mg PO TID-QID	Extensive use in pregnancy is reassuring. Usually combined with APAP or ASA. Habit forming. Limit use near delivery due to fetal respiratory depression.
Methadone (Dolophine)	C	2.5–10 mg PO TID-QID	Limited clinical experience in pregnancy. Variable half life. Inexpensive. Habit forming. Limit use near delivery due to fetal respiratory depression.
Hydromorphone (Dilaudid)	C	1–4 mg PO QID or 3 mg PR BID Liquid available.	Habit forming. Limit use near delivery due to fetal respiratory depression.

Table 4.4 (continued)

Drug	FDA Class	Dose	Comments
Codeine	C	15–60 mg PO TID-QID	Maternal nausea and constipation. Metabolized to morphine. Habit forming. Limit use near delivery due to fetal respiratory depression.
Tramadol (Ultram, Ultracet)	C	25–100 mg PO TID-QID	Well tolerated. May be combined with APAP. Limited clinical experience in pregnancy. Post-marketing reports of neonatal seizures and withdrawal.
Meperidine (Demerol)	C	50–100 mg PO QID Liquid available	Poorly bioavailable. Sedating. Long-duration active metabolite, nor-meperidine, reduces seizure threshold; therefore, repeated dosing should be avoided. Habit forming. Limit use near delivery due to fetal respiratory depression. American Pain Society and Institute for Safe Medicine Practices recommend that this medication NOT be used.

APAP = acetaminophen, ASA = aspirin, PO = by mouth, PR = rectal, QID = four times daily, SL = sublingual, TID = three times daily.
All drugs should be used as needed, with regular use limited to a maximum of two days per week. Recommendations are based on clinical experience and FDA risk category, due to paucity of adequate or controlled clinical trial data during pregnancy. Extensive clinical experience supports safety of acetaminophen, hydrocodone, and morphine. Meperidine may also be used if needed, although repeated dosing with meperidine should be avoided as this can result in accumulation of nor-meperidine with increased risk for seizure.

Table 4.5 Triptan pregnancy registries

Triptan	Company	Contact
Sumatriptan (Imitrex) Naratriptan (Amerge)	GlaxoSmith Kline	800-336-2176 in North America 910-256-0549 outside of North America
Rizatriptan (Maxalt)	Merck	800-986-8999

be obtained at http://www.fda.gov/womens/registries/registries.html. GlaxoSmith Kline and Merck maintain registries for their triptans (Table 4.5).

> **Pearl for the practitioner:**
> Triptans are FDA risk category C drugs and are generally not recommended routinely during pregnancy. Patients using triptans inadvertently or during early pregnancy before realizing they are pregnant should be encouraged by data from small registries and databases that suggest the likelihood of an adverse fetal outcome related to triptan use during pregnancy is probably very small.

Opioids have limited efficacy in migraine and are generally reserved for migraine rescue therapy. Opioids have a long track record of use for treating a variety of pain complaints during pregnancy and are generally considered to be safe during pregnancy. Short-acting opioids, such as hydrocodone (FDA risk category C), may be used when acetaminophen is ineffective. Codeine (FDA risk category B) is generally less desirable, due to constipating and nauseating effects. While codeine has been linked to increased risk for cleft palate and inguinal hernias, these associations have not been substantiated in large epidemiological studies in Europe and the United States [30,31,32]. Patients using opioids during pregnancy should be frequently and carefully monitored to minimize opioid overuse. Regular use of opioid or non-opioid analgesics 3 or more days per week for at least 6 weeks often results in headache worsening or medication overuse headache. Patients chronically using daily opioids during mid-to-late pregnancy should continue daily opioids for the duration of pregnancy because of the risks of fetal mortality and premature labor associated with intrauterine fetal opioid withdrawal [33].

> **Pearl for the practitioner:**
> Opioids can be safely used during pregnancy as rescue agents for severe headaches. Overuse of opioids is a significant concern and use should be carefully monitored.

Sedatives, such as butalbital combination products (e.g., Fiorinol, Fioricet) and isometheptene mucate combination (Midrin) are occasionally beneficial for infrequent migraines in non-pregnant women. Neither should be used routinely during pregnancy.

Herbal Remedies

Most herbal therapies are used for migraine prevention. Peppermint provides analgesic benefits and topical peppermint oil is effective as an acute headache remedy. A solution of 10 g peppermint oil in alcohol may be applied lightly to the forehead and temples during a headache attack and repeated after 15 and 30 minutes. In one study, topical peppermint oil reduced tension-type headache pain by 19% after 30 minutes and 34% after one hour [34]. Although not specifically tested for other headaches, topical peppermint oil may also be worth trying for acute migraines.

Topical preparations are considered likely to be safe during pregnancy [35]. Peppermint oil can only be used as a topical agent and should not be taken internally. Peppermint oil should never be applied to the faces of infants or small children, as this may result in glottal or bronchial spasm and respiratory distress. Therefore, women should be cautioned if they use peppermint oil around babies or toddlers.

> **Pearl for the practitioner:**
> Topical peppermint oil may help reduce acute headache pain. It should not be used around babies or toddlers.

Determining First-Line Migraine Medication Treatment

Several general principles guide prescribing medications to pregnant women:

1. If you don't prescribe a treatment regimen, most women will self-medicate during pregnancy. Initiate communication about safer and effective treatment strategies during the first pregnancy discussion, even if headaches do not seem to be problematic at that time.
2. Limit treatment to FDA risk category A-C medications, selecting A or B treatments when possible.
3. Medication should be recommended at the lowest effective dose, for the shortest possible time, and delayed as long in the pregnancy as possible.

Figure 4.7 provides an algorithm for the treatment of moderate-to-severe migraine.

Prednisone is an FDA risk category B drug, and may be used as rescue therapy when acute treatment has failed and disabling migraine is prolonged

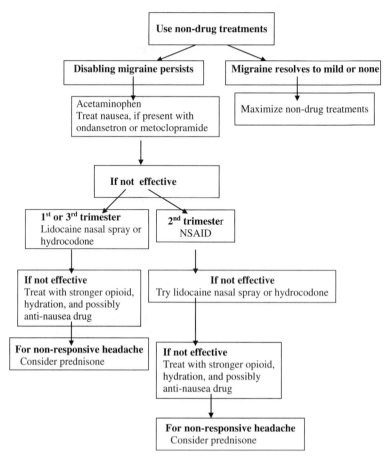

Fig. 4.7 Recommendations for treatment of migraine during conception and pregnancy

and unremitting. In non-pregnant patients, tapering oral doses of steroids over four days (e.g., prednisone 80 mg initially, reduced by 20 mg each day) is reported to be beneficial for unremitting, severe migraine [36]. Another treatment regimen that can be recommended is a short course of prednisone—20 mg twice daily for 5 days. Prednisone is preferred over dexamethasone because the latter crosses the placenta much more readily.

Effectively Communicating Medication Advice

Healthcare providers often feel too rushed during patient appointments to effectively communicate diagnostic impressions and treatment recommendations, as well as address patient concerns. Stresses associated with the patient

Table 4.6 Doctor-patient miscommunications

What the doctor says	What the doctor means	What the patient hears
Your headaches are only migraines.	You don't have a brain tumor and nothing's wrong with your pregnancy.	Why are you complaining about such a minor problem?
Migraines usually improve during pregnancy.	We can probably use safer treatments to effectively treat your milder headaches during your pregnancy.	Don't treat the headaches— they're going to go away on their own anyway.
I'm not going to prescribe anything for your mild or moderate migraines.	Use non-drug treatments for mild-moderate migraine. These are usually very effective.	When you get a migraine, you'll have to just tough it out with no treatment for nine months.
Besides the headache, are you having problems with nausea?	If nausea is a problem, we need to treat that to minimize migraine-related disability.	Let's talk about something other than your silly headaches!
Let me know how your migraines are doing.	Keep daily diaries and we'll review them at your next visit.	I sure hope you forget to talk about headaches by your next visit.

role often result in patients forgetting to discuss important concerns or clarify misunderstood information, leading to miscommunication. A typical example of doctor-patient miscommunication about acute migraine treatment is described in Table 4.6.

Both healthcare providers and patients need to understand that only a limited amount of information can be communicated during any given visit. Patients report their optimal visit length would be 15 minutes [37]. Interestingly, data from the National Ambulatory Medical Care survey showed that the average primary care appointment lasted 16 minutes [38]. Increasing the time of an office visit is usually not possible for the healthcare provider and not necessarily considered desirable by the patient, who can become easily overwhelmed when presented with too much material in a single visit. Patient handouts are good tools to fill in information gaps and reinforce messages presented during appointments. Written materials can be read and reviewed many times outside of the visit to reinforce the key concepts highlighted during the office visit. Handouts can effectively communicate information to patients, providing them with information to reference when an acute migraine develops. A variety of useful handouts are included in the CD that accompanies this book and in Chapter 10.

A survey of 688 migraineurs ranked desirable physician attributes for the doctor caring for their headaches [39]. The top traits, in descending order, were: willing to answer questions, teaches about treatment, educates about headache causes, and teaches avoidance techniques. Healthcare providers should incorporate these attributes to meet goals for each visit, ensuring that the patient understands:

- Her headache diagnosis;
- What therapies have been recommended and which should be avoided;
- How to monitor progress and that her healthcare provider will be checking on her treatment success;
- When to return for follow-up;
- What symptoms should precipitate an early follow-up or contact with the clinic.

Patients are generally reassured and comforted when their healthcare provider clearly states that he or she will continue to address and monitor the patient for as long as necessary.

Providing patients with safer medication options should include discussions of both prescription and non-prescription medications. Patients failing to secure adequate treatment recommendations may turn to alternative and potentially unreliable resources. Practitioners unfamiliar with safer treatments during pregnancy might also provide undesirable advice. A surprising survey asked French pharmacists for treatment recommendations for several case scenarios, including pregnancy-related headache [40]. Although NSAIDs are generally restricted during the third trimester, 8.5% of pharmacists recommended that a woman in her third trimester use a product including an NSAID. It is imperative for clinicians to develop a specific, clearly written treatment regimen with the patient to give them a step-by-step plan to use to treat their acute headaches. This should help to minimize the need for the patient to consider treatment options that have not been recommended by their healthcare provider.

> **Pearl for the practitioner:**
> Clear written information summarizing office discussions is an excellent way to improve compliance. Explicitly outlining a step-wise treatment strategy helps develop a consistent approach to headache treatment.

Regularly Assess Treatment Efficacy

After receiving recommendations for changes in acute headache treatment, a phone or face-to-face follow-up should be arranged to assess treatment response. Without scheduled follow-up, women often abandon restrictions and resume previous attempts to control migraines with OTC therapies.

Daily headache diaries are effective tools to keep patients focused on treatment recommendations and to provide valuable information about headache activity (Fig. 4.8). Patients should record headache activity and behaviors every day for

Time of Day	Severity						Medications
	0	1	2	3	4	5	
Morning **Record wake time:**							
Noon							
Evening							
Bedtime **Record bed time:**							

List non-medication treatment strategies used:

Did you eat meals and snacks (check if yes):
- ☐ Breakfast
- ☐ Mid-morning snack
- ☐ Lunch
- ☐ Mid-morning snack
- ☐ Dinner
- ☐ Evening snack

Check a box each time you drink 8-ouncs of water:

☐ ☐ ☐ ☐ ☐ ☐ ☐ ☐ ☐ ☐

List today's aerobic exercise:

Fig. 4.8 Daily headache diary

2–4 weeks to assess efficacy of acute therapy. Response can be evaluated sooner in patients with more frequent headache episodes. Patients will need to record headache severity several times daily to provide information about peak pain severity and headache duration. Reviewing diaries should provide information about:

- Compliance with medication recommendations;
- Compliance with non-drug treatments;
- Headache frequency, severity, and duration;
- Possibility of additional headaches, like co-existing tension-type or medication overuse headaches;
- Need for additional preventive therapy.

> ***Pearl for the practitioner:***
> Daily headache diaries are effective tools for collecting complete headache information. Clinicians can readily identify headache patterns when reviewing diaries.

Patients should be seen or contacted two to four weeks after receiving acute treatment recommendations to ensure benefit. Patients using OTC or pre-scribed medication can complete the Acute Migraine Medication Quiz to help identify treatment benefit and areas of inadequate response (Box 4.2). Coupling written instructions with daily headache diaries ensures accurate identification of treatment response.

Box 4.2 Acute migraine medication quiz (Reprinted with permission by New Harbinger Publications, Inc. *10 Simple Solutions for Migraines*, Dawn A. Marcus. www.newharbinger.com)

1. Two hours after taking your acute migraine medication, do you still have substantial pain, sensitivity to light and sound, or nausea?
2. Do you usually need to take two or more doses before the pain goes away?
3. Do you use some acute migraine medication three or more days every week?
4. Do you use over-the-counter painkillers for your headache almost every day?
5. Do your friends, family, or doctors worry that you're overusing your migraine medication?

If you answered "yes" to any of these questions, you are probably not achieving optimal relief from your current migraine medications. Talk to your doctor about a change in therapy.

Scheduling Follow-Up Visits

During early pregnancy, patients with recurrent headaches should be seen more frequently, usually around every 2–4 weeks. More frequent visits during this typically more difficult time can allow the practitioner to assess the course of headaches, the disability associated with the headaches, the efficacy of medica-tions, and concerns that the newly pregnant woman may have. More frequent visits early on also may serve to identify and appropriately attend to the development of medication overuse headaches.

As the pregnancy progresses, visits can become less frequent, particularly if headaches improve, as they do in many patients. A typical schedule is detailed below:

- Non-pregnant women: visits every 3–12 months depending on headache pattern, disability, and co-morbidities. Include preconception planning.
- Pregnant women: first visit as soon as pregnancy is identified to discuss treatment strategies, safer use of medications, non-drug options, and expected headache course during pregnancy.

- First trimester: every 2–4 weeks;
- Second and third trimesters: every 4 weeks unless headaches have significantly improved.
- Postpartum: first visit as soon as feasible after delivery to discuss modifications in the treatment strategy, considering whether the patient intends to breastfeed or not.

Summary

Migraines are typically more frequent and problematic in the first trimester when estrogen levels are changing most dramatically. Because headaches and nausea can be quite severe, many women become frustrated and will choose to self-medicate unless they are counseled otherwise. Even though many practitioners are apprehensive about prescribing medications to pregnant women, there are safer, effective options available. An explicit, thoughtful, written treatment strategy can be very beneficial for lessening the burden of headache episodes. The guiding principles of headache treatment include not treating mild headache episodes with medications, treating nausea aggressively, maximizing non-drug approaches, and if medications are needed, using the lowest dose of the safest medication for the shortest period of time as late in the pregnancy as possible. These principles can significantly help to reduce the burden of suffering and ensure the best safety during pregnancy.

Practical pointers:

- After excluding prenatal vitamins and iron, a majority of pregnant women will use prescription and over-the-counter drugs during their pregnancies—most frequently analgesics and anti-emetics.
- All fertile women should be counseled about expected headache changes and safer treatment options with pregnancy.
- Nausea should be treated with herbal/nutritional therapies, acupressure, or safe anti-emetics.
- Obstetricians most commonly treat nausea during pregnancy with vitamin B6, ginger, promethazine, and ondansetron. Ondansetron and metoclopramide are rated FDA risk category B and promethazine is FDA risk category C.
- Mild headaches may be effectively treated with non-pharmacologic therapies.
- Acute headache medications are designed to supplement rather than replace non-drug pain-relieving techniques.
- Without direction, most women will self-medicate during pregnancy. Discussions of safer and effective treatment strategies should occur

before pregnancy and again during the first pregnancy visit, even if headaches do not seem to be problematic at that time.
- First-line acute medication treatment during pregnancy is acetaminophen. Caffeine may be added to boost analgesic potency.
- Lidocaine nasal spray is a safe alternative acute medication option, although it will usually need to be compounded.
- NSAIDs should be restricted to the second trimester.
- Opioids can be used infrequently as rescue therapy, limiting treatment to no more than 2 days per week to minimize the risk for developing medication overuse headache.
- Pregnant patients should be followed every 2–4 weeks during early pregnancy to monitor headache activity and make necessary treatment adjustments.

References

1. Refuerzo JS, Blackwell SC, Sokol RJ, et al. Use of over-the-counter medications and herbal remedies in pregnancy. *Am J Perinatology* 2005;22:321–324.
2. Lee E, Maneno MK, Smith L, et al. National patterns of medication use during pregnancy. *Pharmacoepid Drug Saf* 2006;15:537–545.
3. Henry A, Crowther C. Patterns of medication use during and prior to pregnancy: the MAP study. *Aust N Z J Obstet Gynaecol* 2000;40:165–172.
4. Coad J, Al-Rasasi B, Morgan J. Nutrient insult in early pregnancy. *Proc Nutr Soc* 2002;61:51–59.
5. Power ML, Milligan LA, Schulkin J. Managing nausea and vomiting of pregnancy: a survey of obstetrician-gynecologists. *J Reprod Med* 2007;52:922–928.
6. American College of Obstetricians and Gynecologists. ACOG practice bulletin #52: nausea and vomiting of pregnancy. *Obstet Gynecol* 2004;103:803–815.
7. Borrelli F, Capasso R, Aviello G, Pittler MH, Izzo AA. Effectiveness and safety of ginger in the treatment of pregnancy-induced nausea and vomiting. *Obstet Gynecol* 2005;105:849–856.
8. Chittumma P, Kaewkiattikun K, Wiriyasiriwach B. Comparison of the effectiveness of ginger and vitamin B6 for treatment of nausea and vomiting in early pregnancy: a randomized double-blind controlled trial. *J Med Assoc Thai* 2007;90:15–20.
9. Smith C, Crowther C, Willson K, Hotham N, McMillian V. A randomized controlled trial of ginger to treat nausea and vomiting in pregnancy. *Obstet Gynecol* 2004;103:639–645.
10. Chuang C, Doyle P, Wang J, et al. Herbal medicines used during the first trimester and major congenital malformations. An analysis of data from a pregnancy cohort study. *Drug Saf* 2006;29:537–548.
11. Bsat FA, Hoffman DE, Seubert DE. Comparison of three outpatient regimens in the management of nausea and vomiting in pregnancy. *J Perinatol* 2003;23:531–535.
12. Marcus DA. Nonpharmacologic treatment of migraine. *TEN* 2001;3:50–55.
13. Gesch D, Bernhardt O, Alte D, et al. Prevalence of signs and symptoms of temporomandibular disorders in an urban and rural German population: results of a population-based Study of Health in Pomerania. *Quintessence Int* 2004;35:143–150.

14. Ballegaard V, Thede-Schmidt-Hansen P, Svensson P, Jensen R. Are headache and temporomandibular disorders related? A blind study. *Cephalalgia* 2008;28:832–841.
15. Turk DC, Zaki HS, Rudy TE. Effects of intraoral appliance and biofeedback/stress management alone and in combination in treating pain and depression in patients with temporomandibular disorders. *J Prosthet Dent* 1993;70:158–164.
16. Lipton RB, Scher AI, Steiner TJ, Bigal ME, Kolodner K, Lieberman JN, Stewart WF. Patterns of health care utilization for migraine in England and the United States. *Neurology* 2003;60:441–448.
17. Streissguth AP, Treder RP, Barr HM, et al. Aspirin and acetaminophen use by pregnant women and subsequent child IQ and attention decrements. *Teratology* 1987;35: 211–219.
18. Li DK, Liu L, Odouli R. Exposure to non-steroidal anti-inflammatory drugs during pregnancy and risk of miscarriage: population based cohort study. *BMJ* 2003; 327:368.
19. Evers S, Áfra J, Frese A, et al. EFNS guideline on the drug treatment of migraine – report of an EFNS task force. *Eur J Neurol* 2006;13:560–572.
20. Kozer E, Nikfar S, Costei A, et al. Aspirin consumption during the first trimester of pregnancy and congenital anomalies: a meta-analysis. *Am J Obstet Gynecol* 2002;187:1623–1630.
21. Nørgard B, Puhé E, Caeizel AE, Skriver MV, Sørensen HT. Aspirin use during early pregnancy and the risk of congenital abnormalities: a population-based case-control study. *Am J Obstet Gynecol* 2005;192:922–923.
22. Klebanoff MA, Berendes HW. Aspirin exposure during the first 20 weeks of gestation and IQ at four years of age. *Teratology* 1988;437:249–255.
23. Peroutka SJ, Lyon JA, Swarbrick J, Liption RB, Kolodner K, Goldstein J. Efficacy of diclofenac sodium softgel 100 mg with or without caffeine 100 mg in migraine without aura: a randomized, double-blind, crossover study. *Headache* 2004;44:136–141.
24. Browne ML. Maternal exposure to caffeine and risk of congenital anomalies: a systematic review. *Epidemiology* 2006;17:324–331.
25. Browne ML, Bell EM, Druschel CM, et al. Maternal caffeine consumption and risk of cardiovascular malformations. *Birth Defects Res A Clin Mol Teratol* 2007;79:533–543.
26. Maizels M, Scott B, Cohen W, Chen W. Intranasal lidocaine for treatment of migraine: a randomized, double-blind, controlled trial. *JAMA* 1996;276:319–321.
27. Soldin OP, Dahlin J, O'Mara DM. Triptans in pregnancy. *Ther Drug Monit* 2008; 30:5–9.
28. Kallen B, Lygner PE. Delivery outcome in women who used drugs for migraine during pregnancy with special reference to sumatriptan. *Headache* 2001;41:351–356.
29. Evans EW, Lorber KC. Use of 5-HT$_1$ agonists in pregnancy. *Ann Pharmacother* 2008;42:543–549.
30. Bracken MB, Holfod TR. Exposure to prescribed drugs in pregnancy and association with congenital malformations. *ObstetGynecol* 1981;58:336–344.
31. Saxén I. Epidemiology of cleft lip and palate. An attempt to rule out chance correlations. *Br J Prev Soc Med* 1875;29:103–110.
32. Saxén I. Associations between oral clefts and drugs taken during pregnancy. *Int J Epidemilol* 1975;4:37–44.
33. Beers MH, Berkow R, eds. Drug use and dependence. The Merck Manual of Diagnostics and Therapeutics, 17th edition, Section 15, Chapter 195. (Available at www.merck.com/pubs Accessed September 30, 2007.)
34. Göbel H, Fresenius J, Heinze A, Dworschak M, Soyka D. Effectiveness of Oleum menthae piperitae and paracetamol in therapy of headache of the tension type. *Nervenarzt* 1996;67:672–681.

35. Kligler B, Chaudhary S. Peppermint oil. *Am Fam Physician* 2007;75:1027–1030.
36. Von Seggern RL, Adelman JU. Practice and economics cost considerations in headache treatment. Part 2: acute migraine treatment. *Headache* 1996;36:493–502.
37. Landau DA, Bachner YG, Elishkewitz K, Goldstein L, Barneboim E. Patients' views on optimal visit length in primary care. *J Med Pract Manage* 2007;23:12–15.
38. Woodwell DA, Cherry DK. National Ambulatory Medical Care Survey: 2002 summary. *Adv Data* 2004;26:1–44.
39. Lipton RB, Stewart WF. Acute migraine therapy: do doctors understand what patients with migraine want from therapy? *Headache* 1999;39(Suppl 2):S20–S26.
40. Damase-Michel C, Vié C, Lacroix I, Lapeyre-Mestre M, Montastruc JL. Drug counselling in pregnancy: an opinion survey of French community pharmacists. *Pharmacoepidemiol Drug Saf* 2004;13:711–715.

Chapter 5
Acute Treatment Options for the Lactating Headache Patient

Key Chapter Points

- While headaches often decrease during the second and third trimesters, they usually recur postpartum. Fatigue, interrupted sleep, changes in routine, and decreased estradiol levels can all result in a lowered headache threshold and more headaches.
- Common secondary causes of postpartum headache include pre-eclampsia/eclampsia, post-procedural low pressure spinal headache, and cerebral venous thrombosis.
- Breastfeeding should be encouraged for the myriad of health benefits for the infant and mother and because headaches are often attenuated in the breast-feeding mother.
- Safer, effective treatment options for pain and nausea are available to the breastfeeding mother.
- Non-pharmacological therapies should be used for mild-to-moderate severity headaches.
- Preferred acute medications for lactating women treating headaches are acetaminophen, ibuprofen, and sumatriptan. The preferred medication for nausea is ondansetron.
- Opioids may be used in single doses, monitoring the baby for side effects.

Keywords American Academy of Pediatrics · Breastfeeding · Nursing · Postpartum · World Health Organization

Katie is a 26-year-old who delivered a healthy term baby two weeks ago: "I was so thrilled when I was pregnant to have my migraines gone! I'd really forgotten how bad my headaches could get until I went home after Justin was born and started getting headaches about a week later. I wasn't sure what to do for the pain, but I have some old Imitrex from before I was pregnant that I used. I didn't know if this would be safe for Justin, so I briefly stopped nursing and wonder if I should just switch to bottle feeding." Katie's primary care provider assured her that she could still treat her headaches and nurse the baby, providing her with an effective treatment strategy to use during lactation. Katie was able to successfully control her headaches and continued breastfeeding for nine months.

D.A. Marcus, P.A. Bain, *Effective Migraine Treatment in Pregnant and Lactating Women: A Practical Guide*, DOI 10.1007/978-1-60327-439-5_5, © Humana Press, a part of Springer Science+Business Media, LLC 2009

Proactive discussions during the third trimester about plans for headache management after delivery can help provide patients like Katie with a better understanding about headache expectations and safer treatments to be used when nursing. As described in Chapter 2, breastfeeding should be encouraged due to the numerous health benefits for both baby and mother.

Fortunately, the majority of women begin feeding their babies using breast milk. Although chronic headaches improve in the second and third trimesters of pregnancy in the majority of women, they usually recur postpartum. As noted in Chapter 2, return of headaches after delivery is often delayed in women who choose to breastfeed. Nursing mothers, therefore, should be encouraged to breastfeed and should receive counseling about safer medication regimens while nursing. The good news for patients is that medication treatment options increase after delivery, although some restrictions are still necessary. Several principles guide the acute treatment of headaches in the lactating patient:

- Consider important secondary causes of headache.
- Anticipate headache recurrence after delivery.
- Develop a safer and effective acute treatment plan.

Consider Important Secondary Causes of Headache

Postpartum headaches are commonly caused by primary headaches, such as migraine and tension-type headache. A prospective study evaluating 985 women delivering over a three-month assessment period identified postpartum headache in 39% of women [1]. Median time to onset of headache was two days after delivery. Diagnostic etiologies for these postpartum headaches are shown in Fig. 5.1, with two in three headaches attributed to migraine or tension-type

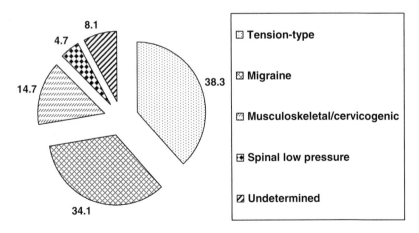

Fig. 5.1 Causes of early postpartum headache (Based on [1])

headaches. A recent, retrospective review of 95 patients hospitalized for severe, later onset postpartum headache beginning >24 hours after delivery also identified tension-type headache as the most common individual cause of severe headache (Fig. 5.2) [2].

Although postpartum headaches are often caused by tension-type headache or migraine recurrence, secondary causes of headache must be considered (Table 5.1). While central venous thrombosis and low pressure headache after anesthesia are generally considered in the differential diagnosis of postpartum headache, pre-eclampsia/eclampsia is often overlooked, particularly when occurring after the immediate post-delivery period. In a review of all cases of eclampsia seen during a five-year period ($N = 89$), one in three cases occurred postpartum [3]. Postpartum diagnoses occurred up to 14 days after delivery, with 79% of postpartum diagnoses made >48 hours after giving birth. In comparison to women diagnosed before delivery or within 48 hours after delivery, women with late-onset postpartum eclampsia (>48 hours after delivery) were more likely to have experienced headache (odds ratio = 4.1), visual symptoms (odds ratio = 2.6), or at least one symptom of pre-eclampsia [e.g., persistent headaches, blurred vision, epigastric pain, nausea, or vomiting] (odds ratio = 4.6). Among women experiencing symptoms of pre-eclampsia, only one in three sought medical attention, with the majority not seeking medical care because they did not consider their symptom(s) to be serious. This study highlights the need to be vigilant for pre-eclampsia and eclampsia during the first 2 weeks postpartum and the need to specifically seek information on the occurrence of pre-eclampsia symptoms to avoid eclampsia when possible. Recently, an analysis of 10 case reports of postpartum eclampsia reported symptoms occurring on average on day 8 after delivery, with a range of 4–11 days postpartum [4]. Visual changes occurred in 60% of cases, including scotoma (blind spots), blurred vision, and blindness. Spinal fluid analysis was

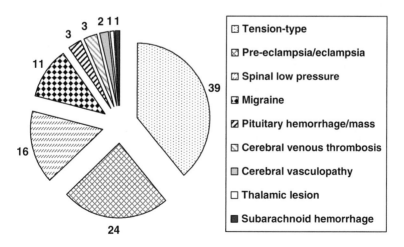

Fig. 5.2 Etiology of severe headache occurring >24 hours postpartum (Based on [2])

Table 5.1 Secondary postpartum headaches

Condition	Risk Factors	Typical Time Course	Diagnostic features	Testing abnormalities
Central venous thrombosis	Dehydration, infection, hypercoagulable	1st two postpartum weeks	Papilledema, change in mental status, seizure	Abnormal MRI or MR venogram
Low pressure headache	Epidural or spinal anesthesia	1st postpartum week	Postural headache	Opening spinal pressure <120 mm H_2O
Pre-eclampsia, Eclampsia	Nulliparous, carrying more than one baby, age >35 years old, obesity, gestational diabetes, history of pre-eclampsia	1st two postpartum weeks	Hypertension, proteinuria, seizure	MRI, CT, and arteriography evidence of vasospasm and edema. Spinal fluid may show elevated cells and protein.
Intracranial hemorrhage, cerebrovascular accident	Cardiovascular risk factors, trauma, systemic Lupus erythematosus	Variable	Focal neurological symptoms/signs, altered mental status	MRI or CT evidence of bleeding or ischemia. Spinal fluid analysis for blood or xanthochromia
Meningitis	Epidural/spinal anesthesia Possibly episiotomy	Variable	Fever, neck stiffness, photophobia, focal neurological symptoms/signs, altered mental status	Inflammatory and infectious changes on spinal fluid evaluation
Infrequent causes of postpartum headache				
Pituitary apoplexy	Anticoagulant use or coagulopathy Head trauma Surgery	Abrupt course: developing over 1–2 days	Sudden onset of severe headache, nausea, visual disturbance, fever, neck stiffness	Abnormal MRI

Table 5.1 (continued)

Condition	Risk Factors	Typical Time Course	Diagnostic features	Testing abnormalities
Intracranial tumor	Growth of pre-existing pituitary adenomas and meningiomas may be accelerated during pregnancy	Slowly progressive development of headache and neurological symptoms	Neurological complaints, depending on tumor location	Abnormal MRI
Benign intracranial hypertension (pseudotumor cerebri)	Obesity Treatment with tetracycline, lithium, corticosteroids, or vitamin A	Gradual development of symptoms	Diffuse, constant headache, papilledema, sixth nerve palsy, visual obscurations*	Opening spinal pressure >250 mm H_2O
Carotid dissection	Hypertension Neck manipulation or trauma	Abrupt onset, worsens over 1–2 days	Neck pain radiating to the jaw Focal neurological deficits Ptosis with miosis	Abnormal MR angiogram

CT = computed tomography; MR = magnetic resonance; MRI = magnetic resonance imaging
*Visual obscurations are episodes of temporary blindness typically lasting <1 minute associated with increased intracranial pressure. Characteristically occurs when rising from sitting to standing position.

performed in seven patients, with elevated cell counts and protein in four patients. Magnetic resonance imaging showed cerebral changes in 60% of patients, with abnormalities in some patients on computed tomography and arteriography. The diagnosis of eclampsia/pre-eclampsia usually is suggested when the patient presents with headache, hypertension, proteinuria, and/or seizures.

> *Pearl for the practitioner:*
> Secondary headaches should be considered in women with headaches occurring after delivery. Pre-eclampsia and eclampsia are often overlooked as a possible secondary cause of postpartum headache.

The risk for meningitis may be slightly increased after delivery due to spinal and epidural anesthetic procedures [5] and secondary bacteremia from vaginal contamination. Meningitis after delivery or spinal anesthesia, however, is quite rare. For example, only 13 cases of postpartum group B streptococcal meningitis have been reported in the literature, with a few possibly caused by secondary bacteria from an episiotomy or vaginal lacerations [6]. Nevertheless, meningitis should be considered in the postpartum patient, especially if fever, nuchal rigidity, and nausea and vomiting are present. Recommendations for the evaluation for possible secondary headaches are provided in Chapter 9.

> *Pearl for the practitioner:*
> While the vast majority of postpartum headaches are tension-type and migraine, the clinician should be ever vigilant for the less common, but ominous secondary causes of headache.

Though tension-type headache and migraine recurrence are common causes of headache after delivery, clinicians must be vigilant about less common, but more ominous types of headaches. The threshold for further investigation, including physical examination, laboratory testing, and possibly neuroimaging, should be low for women with new or severe headaches following delivery because of the potentially devastating consequences of a missed diagnosis.

Anticipate Headache Recurrence After Delivery

While clinicians and women should be encouraged by headache reduction or remission during pregnancy, patients should be counseled that chronic headaches, including migraine, typically recur after delivery. Failure to alert patients to the likely return of headache may result in unnecessary concerns when headaches do recur and prevent adequate availability of acute therapies, especially after mom has returned home. The postpartum period can be particularly stressful: adjusting to having a new family member, changes in daily routines, and alterations in sleeping patterns. Discussions about likely changes in headache activity and safer treatment options after delivery will help reduce maternal anxiety and frustration and minimize risk for erratically treated headaches.

Patients should be encouraged to breastfeed because of numerous benefits for the baby and the likelihood of delayed migraine recurrence in women choosing to nurse. An Italian study prospectively followed 49 women with active migraine during pregnancy and postpartum [7]. The number of migraine attacks in study participants decreased 58% from the first to second trimester and 82% from the first to third trimester. By the third trimester, migraine remission had occurred in 79% of women. After delivery, headache recurrence was significantly affected by breastfeeding ($P<0.001$), with increased likelihood of migraine recurrence after both one week and one month among women choosing to bottle feed (Fig. 5.3). Therefore, breastfeeding tends to delay the return of headaches to pre-pregnancy patterns.

Patients should receive information that:

- Migraines will likely recur during the first 1–4 weeks after delivery.
- Breastfeeding is apt to postpone the return of migraines.
- Nursing is not expected to aggravate chronic headaches.
- Medication restrictions will be necessary while nursing:
  - Acute treatments (except for anti-emetics) that were safe during pregnancy can generally be used while breastfeeding;
  - Some acute treatments that were restricted during pregnancy will be available for use when nursing.

> **Pearl for the practitioner:**
> Women should be encouraged to breastfeed because of numerous benefits for infant and mother, including delayed headache recurrence.

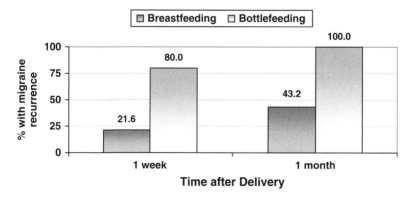

Fig. 5.3 Effect of breastfeeding on postpartum migraine recurrence (Based on [7])

Utilize Good Principles of Acute Headache Treatment

As detailed in Chapter 4, acute headache medications can be appropriate for infrequent, moderate-to-severe headaches. The same principles that govern the use of acute therapy during pregnancy also apply when nursing:

- Maximize use of non-drug treatments:
  - Relaxation and biofeedback;
  - Cognitive restructuring;
  - Distraction techniques;
  - Stretching exercises;
  - Heat and ice;
  - Acupressure;
  - Sleep.
- Reserve acute medications for moderate-to-severe headaches to minimize the risk of developing medication overuse (rebound) headaches.
- Limit regular use of acute medications to no more than two days per week;
  - Avoid repeat dosing for the same headache, if possible.
- Select the safest effective medications.
- Maintain headache diaries to monitor medication effectiveness and usage patterns.

Select the Safest Medications

In general, headache medications (with the exception of some anti-emetics used as adjunctive headache treatment) that were safe to use during pregnancy are usually safe when nursing. The primary issue is the amount of medication that appears in the milk and expectations for side effects in the nursing baby with typical maternal drug doses. A review of factors affecting drug safety during lactation is detailed in Chapter 2. Medication selection for the nursing mother should be guided by several principles to maximize safer use of effective therapy:

- Choose medications that:
  - Have limited risk to the baby:
    - Are safe to use directly by the baby (may be age dependent);
    - Are considered to be safe during breastfeeding by reliable sources;
    - For which extensive data regarding use in baby or with nursing are available;
  - Result in a low concentration in mother's milk:
    - Low oral bioavailability;
    - High protein binding;
    - Low lipid solubility;

- High molecular weight;
- Short half-life;

- Minimize baby's exposure by:
  - Using the lowest effective dose;
  - Avoiding repeated dosing;
  - Timing maternal medication administration to minimize baby's risk.

Time Maternal Medication Dosing

Immediately following delivery, milk production is quite low for the first 1–2 days after delivery and medications given at this time are unlikely to be present in sufficient amounts to affect the newborn. After the first few days, when milk production increases, the issue of mother-to-infant transfer of medications becomes more important. Maternal medication usage, therefore, becomes a greater concern after this immediate postpartum period. Certain medications can be given to the infant without regard to timing of ingestion, such as acetaminophen (safe for infant) and ibuprofen (minimal amount appears in the breast milk).

The administration of maternal medications should ideally be timed to minimize exposure to the baby. In cases where acute medications that require cautious use need to be used to manage severe acute attacks, mom may wish to pump and store extra breast milk on days when she has not used medications (Box 5.1). This milk might then be used on days when maternal medication exposure is necessary. Drug exposure to the nursing baby can be minimized by administering medications immediately after completing breastfeeding, allowing the ingested drug to be metabolized and excreted before the next breastfeeding session. If non-compatible drugs are used between feedings, breast milk might be expressed and discarded for several hours after dosing, supplementing feeds with stored milk.

Box 5.1 Storing breast milk

- Always wash your hands before expressing milk
- Choosing a container for breast milk
  - Use sealable container, such as bottle with screw top
  - Wash container with soapy water or clean in dishwasher before use
  - Use plastic when using within a few hours or refrigerating
  - Use glass when freezing
  - Do not store in disposable bottle liners

- Amount to put in individual container
  - Store as 2–4 ounce portions (¼–½ cup)
  - May use clean ice cube tray for storage—each cube is about 1 ounce. Cover tray while storing milk.

- Acceptable duration of storage of freshly expressed milk
  - Up to 10 hours at room temperature
  - Up to 24 hours in cooler with ice packs
  - Up to 1 week in refrigerator
    - Store in back of refrigerator rather than on door to achieve better maintained temperature
  - Up to 2 weeks in freezer
    - Thaw 12 hours in refrigerator
    - Never microwave
    - May refrigerate for 24 hours after thawing
    - Do not re-freeze
  - Resources for more information
    - http://www.llli.org/nb.html [La Leche League International website]
    - http://www.breastfeed-essentials.com/storagehandling.html
    - http://www.breastfeedingbasics.com

Specific Medication Recommendations

Both the American Academy of Pediatrics (http://aappolicy.aappublications. org/) and the World Health Organization (WHO; http://www.who.int/child-adolescent-health/) provide online resources cataloguing drug safety. Table 5.2 divides acute medication categories, using information provided by both organizations. Only some drugs within any drug category are listed, due to the availability of literature to make safety determinations. Furthermore, the WHO's recommendations note that drug safety may depend on the age of the nursing baby, with the capacity to absorb and eliminate drugs different in premature infants and newborns in comparison with older babies. In general, extra caution should be exercised when administering drugs to nursing mothers of premature babies or infants <1 month old. Additional resources cataloguing safe medication usage during nursing are detailed in Chapter 2. Another excellent resource is *Medications and Mother's Milk* by Dr. Thomas Hale, a noted authority on medication use during breastfeeding.

Analgesics

Acetaminophen (Tylenol) and ibuprofen (Motrin) are preferred analgesics when breastfeeding. Ibuprofen is generally more effective as a headache remedy. Ibuprofen has poor transfer to milk [8] and its use in children is well documented. Other non-steroidal anti-inflammatory drugs (NSAIDs; e.g., naproxen [Naprosyn, Aleve], piroxicam [Feldene], and sulindac [Clinoril]) are excreted into the

Table 5.2 Acute headache medications during lactation

Medication	Dosage	Comments
Compatible with breastfeeding		
Acetaminophen (Tylenol)	325–650 mg PO QID Liquid & PR available	Do not exceed 3.5 g daily
Ibuprofen (Motrin)	400 mg PO TID-QID Liquid available	Take with food
Intranasal lidocaine	4% compounded solution. 0.5–1 mL. May repeat once.	Best studied for cluster headache. May help about half with migraine.
Prednisone	80 mg PO initially, reduced by 20 mg each day for 4 days Or 20 mg twice daily for 5 days	Treatment of status migrainosus (severe migraine persisting >72 hours). Take with food. Wait at least 4 hours to breastfeed to minimize baby's exposure.
Sumatriptan (Imitrex)	25–100 mg PO	Only triptan with adequate data available to determine safety with nursing. No need to pump and discard milk.
Compatible with breastfeeding, use caution*		
Aspirin	650 mg PO	Monitor for hemolysis, increased bleeding, and metabolic acidosis
Butorphanol (Stadol)	Nasal spray or injection for severe, recalcitrant headaches. Monitor for overuse.	Monitor for apnea, bradycardia, and cyanosis. Generally not recommended: high risk for misuse/abuse
Caffeine	100 mg PO added to analgesic	Monitor for irritability and poor sleep. Effects may be prolonged.
Codeine	15–30 mg PO	May result in elevated morphine levels. Monitor for apnea, bradycardia, and cyanosis. Single dose likely safe.
Morphine (MSIR)	10–30 mg PO/PR	Monitor for apnea, bradycardia, and cyanosis. Single dose likely safe.
Naproxen (Naprosyn, Aleve)	250–500 mg PO	Although no known effects, less safety documentation available than for ibuprofen.
Ondansetron (Zofran)	4–8 mg PO BID Liquid and ODT available	Excreted in rodent breast milk; human breast milk concentrations not studied. Preferred anti-emetic during nursing.
Topical peppermint oil	10% peppermint oil in ethanol applied to the forehead	Do not use near babies' or children's faces; can cause serious bucco-oral and bronchial spasms
Avoid if possible		
Ergotamine (Cafergot, Wigraine)	Not recommended	Monitor for infant ergotism

Table 5.2 (continued)

Medication	Dosage	Comments
Metoclopramide (Reglan)	Not recommended	Insufficient data, but possible neural developmental effects
Promethazine (Phenergan)	Not recommended	Black box warning for pediatric use. Manufacturer does not recommend when nursing.
Insufficient data to permit recommendation		
Meclizine (Antivert, Dramamine)	Insufficient data for recommendation	Excretion into human milk unknown. Effects with nursing inadequately studied.
Prochlorperazine (Compazine)	Insufficient data for recommendation	Excreted into human milk. Effects with nursing inadequately studied.

*Avoid repeat dosing and monitor infant for side effects.
BID = twice daily, ODT = orally disintegrating tablet, PO = by mouth, PR = rectal, QID = four times daily, TID = three times daily
All drugs should be used as needed, with regular use limited to a maximum of 2 days per week.

breast milk and have undesirable longer half-lives that may result in drug accumulation with repeat dosing. The American Academy of Pediatrics lists naproxen as compatible with breastfeeding, although data supporting this classification are less abundant than with ibuprofen [9]. Indomethacin is also catalogued as compatible, although a single case of seizure was noted [9].

> *Pearl for the practitioner:*
> Acetaminophen and ibuprofen are preferred first-line treatment options for headache pain when breastfeeding.

While opioids can be considered compatible with breastfeeding when used infrequently and only occasionally, the WHO cautions against repeated doses, with the need to carefully monitor the baby for apnea, bradycardia, and cyanosis. This caution is supported by a case report of an infant dying from a very high serum level of morphine caused by repeated use of acetaminophen plus codeine by a mother who was a cytochrome P450 CYP2D6 ultra-rapid metabolizer [10]. Codeine is metabolized to morphine via CYP2D6 and newborns have a reduced capacity to metabolize and eliminate morphine. Duplications of CYP2D6 genes can result in ultra-rapid drug metabolism and have been demonstrated in 1.3% of Caucasian Americans, 5.8% of African-Americans, and 2.0% of racially mixed Americans [11]. The occurrence of rapid metabolizers among a minority of breastfeeding mothers would result in an increased requirement for codeine in these patients to achieve the analgesic effect and exposure of unexpectedly high morphine concentrations to their breastfed infants. For this reason, repeated dosing should be minimized.

> **Pearl for the practitioner:**
> Single doses of opioids are safe. Repeated doses, especially when taken by women who are rapid metabolizers, can be problematic and should be avoided.

Experience with tramadol (Ultram) during nursing is limited. About 0.1% of the maternal tramadol dosage can be recovered in breast milk. Due to the limited information about safety with infant exposure, tramadol is generally not recommended when nursing.

Triptans

Sumatriptan was the first triptan developed as acute migraine-specific therapy. Sumatriptan is minimally excreted into breast milk, with only 0.24% of the maternal dosage recovered in breast milk [12]. Although initial recommendations for women using sumatriptan while nursing was to pump and discard milk for several hours after a sumatriptan dose, the American Academy of Pediatrics subsequently determined that sumatriptan is compatible with breastfeeding without needing to pump and discard the milk [9]. Data for other triptans is inadequate to provide safe recommendations.

> **Pearl for the practitioner:**
> Sumatriptan is minimally excreted in breast milk and is considered compatible with breastfeeding.

Rescue Therapy

Status migrainosus is defined as a migraine episode that has failed to respond to acute care therapy after three days. Status migrainosus is typically managed with triptans or dihydroergotamine in non-pregnant, non-nursing patients. Tapering oral doses of prednisone or a short 5-day course of prednisone (e.g., 20 mg twice daily for 5 days) may be used as rescue therapy in patients failing to respond to migraine-specific drugs or analgesics [13]. Steroids are not contraindicated during breastfeeding when used in small doses for short periods, as described above. To reduce exposure, wait at least 4 hours after an oral steroid dose before breastfeeding.

Anti-emetics

Since nausea frequently accompanies migraine and is often responsible for a significant amount of the disability associated with the migraine attack, having safer, effective anti-nausea options can be very useful. Data on drug excretion into breast milk and safe use with nursing are limited for most anti-nausea medications. The American Gastroenterological Association recently published literature-based recommendations for the use of anti-emetics during lactation [14]. Among those anti-emetics typically used as adjunctive migraine treatment, limited human data with nursing were available for metoclopramide (Reglan), with no human data for ondansetron (Zofran), prochlorperazine (Compazine), and promethazine (Phenergan). Both metoclopramide and prochlorperazine were considered to have potential toxicity, though metoclopramide has a low milk-to-plasma ratio and is considered the safer of the two. The American Academy of Pediatrics advises that metoclopramide should be used with caution [9]. While ondansetron and promethazine are considered to be probably compatible with breastfeeding, there is concern with promethazine. A black box warning against using promethazine in pediatric patients <2 years old suggests caution with nursing may also be warranted. For this reason, the preferred anti-emetic during lactation is ondansetron.

> *Pearl for the practitioner:*
> Migraine-related nausea should be treated. Ondansetron is the preferred anti-nausea medication for nursing women with nausea.

Herbal Remedies

Dilute, topical peppermint oil (10% peppermint oil in ethanol) has demonstrated benefit for reducing tension-type headaches in non-pregnant persons, with no data available for efficacy with migraine or other headaches [15,16]. Although peppermint oil has not been specifically tested during lactation, dilute, topical peppermint for headache is considered relatively safe during nursing [17,18]. Peppermint oil should never be used near babies' or children's faces, however, as it can induce potentially dangerous bucco-oral and bronchial spasms [17].

Although ginger is recommended to treat pregnancy-related nausea, minimal data are available about the safety of using ginger during lactation. Despite the lack of data, it is believed that ginger is probably compatible with nursing [19].

Summary

Even though headaches usually diminish in the second and third trimesters of pregnancy, they usually recur after delivery. Headache recurrence is postponed by breastfeeding. During the final months of pregnancy, strategies should be developed with the patient for treating returning headaches. Women should be encouraged to inform their clinicians about any change in headache pattern to ensure secondary headaches have not developed. Fortunately, a variety of medications can be safely used to acutely treat headache symptoms when nursing.

> ***Practical pointers:***
>
> - Pre-delivery headache counseling helps plan strategies for the likely return of headaches after the baby is born.
> - Acetaminophen and ibuprofen are safe and effective first-line headache medications. Sumatriptan is a safe, effective second-line treatment for severe headache episodes.
> - Ondansetron is preferred for nausea when nursing.
> - If necessary, single doses of opioids can be used as rescue treatment.
> - Frequent use of acute treatments should prompt consideration for headache prevention therapy.
> - Administration of certain maternal medications should be timed to minimize exposure to the nursing baby.

References

1. Goldszmidt E, Kern R, Chaput A, Macarthur A. The incidence and etiology of postpartum headaches: a prospective cohort study. *Can J Anaesth* 2005;52:971–977.
2. Stella CI, Jodicke CD, How HY, Harkness UF, Sibai BM. Postpartum headache: is your work-up complete? *Am J Obstet Gynecol* 2007;196:318.e1–318.e7.
3. Chames MC, Livingston JC, Ivester TS, Barton JR, Sibai BM. Late postpartum eclampsia: a preventable disease? *Am J Obstet Gynecol* 2002;186:1174–1177.
4. Santos VM, Correa FG, Modesto FR, Moutella PR. Late-onset postpartum eclampsia: still a diagnostic dilemma? *Hong Kong Med J* 2008;14:60–63.
5. Baer ET. Post-dural puncture bacterial meningitis. *Anesthesiology* 2006;105:381–393.
6. Gielchinsky Y, Cohen R, Revel A, Ezra Y. Postpartum maternal group B streptococcal meningitis. *Acta Obstet Gynecol Scand* 2005;84:490–491.
7. Sances G, Granella F, Nappi A, et al. Course of migraine during pregnancy and postpartum: a prospective study. *Cephalalgia* 2003;23:197–205.
8. Davies NM. Clinical pharmacokinetics of ibuprofen. The first 30 years. *Clin Pharmacokinet* 1998;34:101–154.
9. American Academy of Pediatric Committee on Drugs. The transfer of drugs and other chemicals into human milk. *Pediatrics* 2001;108:776–789.
10. Koren G, Cairns J, Chitayat D, Gaedigk A, Leeder SJ. Pharmacogenetics of morphine poisoning in a breastfed neonate of a codeine-prescribed mother. *Lancet* 2006;368:704.
11. Gaedigk A, Ndjontché L, Divakaran K, et al. Cytochrome P4502D6 (CYP2D6) gene locus heterogeneity: characterization of gene duplication events. *Clin Pharmacol Ther* 2007;81:242–251.
12. Wojnar-Horton RE, Hackett LP, Yapp P, et al. Distribution and excretion of sumatriptan in human milk. *Br J Clin Pharmacol* 1996;41:217–221.

13. Von Seggern RL, Adelman JU: Practice and economics cost considerations in headache treatment. Part 2: acute migraine treatment. *Headache* 1996;36:493–502.
14. Mahadevan U, Kane S. American Gastroenterological Association Institute Medical Position Statement on the Use of Gastrointestinal Medications in Pregnancy. *Gastroenterology* 2006;131:283–311.
15. Göbel H, Schmidt G, Soyka D. Effect of peppermint and eucalyptus oil preparations on neurophysiological and experimental algesimetric headache parameters. *Cephalalgia* 1994;14:228–234.
16. Göbel H, Fresenius J, Heinze A, Dworschak M, Soyka D. Effectiveness of Oleum menthae piperitae and paracetamol in therapy of headache of the tension type. *Nervenarzr* 1996;67;672–681.
17. Kliger B, Chaudhary S. Peppermint oil. *Am Fam Physician* 2007;75;1027–1030.
18. Blumenthal M. The ABC clinical guide to herbs. American Botanical Council, Austin, TX, 2003.
19. Briggs GG, Freeman RK, Yaffe SJ. Drugs in pregnancy and lactation: a reference guide to fetal and neonatal risk, 7th ed. Portland, OR, Lippincott Williams & Wilkins, 2005, p. 725.

Chapter 6
Preventive Treatment Options for the Pregnant Headache Patient

Key Chapter Points

- Most pregnant women with headaches note significant improvement in their headache pattern by the end of the first trimester with sustained improvement in the second and third trimesters.
- Patients failing to note improvement by the end of the first trimester generally continue to experience headaches throughout the remainder of pregnancy. These patients may be candidates for preventive therapy.
- Use of safe preventive agents is preferred over allowing the woman to overuse acute pain medications and risk developing medication overuse (analgesic rebound) headaches.
- Non-drug approaches should be considered first and maximized to limit the need for headache preventive medication during pregnancy.
- Safe options for headache preventive therapy, including propranolol, gabapentin in early pregnancy, and magnesium are available.
- Headache prevention medication, if used during pregnancy, requires close cooperation among the headache-treating provider, the patient, and the obstetrician.

Keywords Antidepressant · Antiepileptic · Antihypertensive · Malformation · Prevention

At her doctor visit during the second week of her 2nd trimester, Courtney insists, "Everyone keeps telling me my headaches will get better with pregnancy, so I don't want to take the time to learn biofeedback, since my headaches are going to get better anyway. And I know it's bad to use lots of medications; so I'm just toughing it out until things get better." When Courtney returns in one month, she has lost 2 pounds, which she relates to poor appetite from frequent headaches and nausea. She has been to the emergency room three times for intravenous treatment for dehydration after prolonged headache episodes. She is currently using Tylenol several days per week and an old Vicodin prescription that her husband had in the medicine cabinet. Courtney has been on sick leave from work for the last 3 weeks and has been spending most days lying in bed in tears.

D.A. Marcus, P.A. Bain, *Effective Migraine Treatment in Pregnant and Lactating Women: A Practical Guide*, DOI 10.1007/978-1-60327-439-5_6, © Humana Press, a part of Springer Science+Business Media, LLC 2009

Fortunately, Courtney's story is not typical, because the majority of patients experience headache improvement as their pregnancies progress into the second and third trimesters. Unfortunately, the minority of patients who continue to experience problematic headaches during pregnancy will often suffer with significant disability as they wait in vain for headache relief. Failure to identify and treat frequent and disabling headaches that persist throughout pregnancy can, as in Courtney's case, lead to poor nutrition, dehydration, mood disturbance, disability, and discouragement. It is important to recognize those who would benefit most from preventive therapy during pregnancy early before disability has developed.

Although most patients notice improvement in their headache pattern as the first trimester comes to a close, published data provide the clinician with useful information that can allow him or her to predict which patients will benefit most from preventive treatment. In a longitudinal survey of the natural history of headache during pregnancy, those patients who continued to experience problematic headaches at the end of their first trimester (like Courtney) typically experienced headaches throughout the remainder of their pregnancies (Fig. 6.1) [1]. Fig. 6.2 shows average change in headache activity during the last 6 months of pregnancy and first 3 months after delivery in this study. Headache was quantified using the headache index, a standard measure of headache activity. The headache index was calculated as a mean headache intensity from 4-times daily headache severity diary recordings, with headaches rated at each time point on a 0 (no headache) to 10 (incapacitating headache) scale. Because many recording points represent no headache in most patients

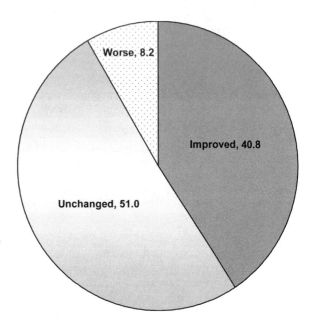

Fig. 6.1 Percentages of patients reporting headache at the end of their first trimester who experience a change in headache during the second or third trimesters (Based on [1])

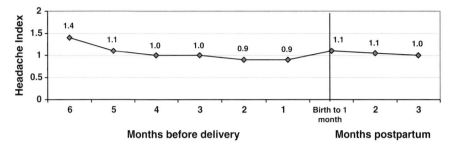

Fig. 6.2 Natural course of headaches during pregnancy. Headache index is an average headache severity score (Based on [1])

Headache index was calculated by adding 4 times daily headache severity scores (rated as 0 = no headache and 10 = severe, disabling headache) and dividing by the number of recorded points. The headache index, therefore, represents an average daily headache score that incorporates headache severity, duration, and frequency. Headache index scores are typically low numbers, as seen here, since any day with no headache would include four scores of zero.

with episodic headache, headache index scores are typically low, as also seen in this study. Headaches improved by only 30% during the 2nd and 3rd trimesters. Therefore, those patients experiencing frequent headaches after the first trimester may be candidates for preventive therapy.

> **Pearl for the practitioner:**
> Most pregnant patients with headaches will notice significant improvement in their headache pattern by the end of the first trimester. It is important to identify those whose headache pattern will not likely improve, as these patients are more apt to benefit from preventive therapy.

Identify Patients Needing Preventive Therapy

Patients should be considered candidates for prevention therapy if their headaches are:

- Frequent:
  - Typically occurring 3 or more days per week;
- Disabling or prolonged:
  - Substantial and consistent loss of social or work activities due to headaches;
  - Associated with poor nutrition or dehydration;
- Not responsive to appropriate acute treatment.

> **Box 6.1** Migraine Prevention Quiz (Reprinted with permission from DA Marcus. *10 Simple Solutions for Migraines*, New Harbinger, Oakland, CA, 2006)
>
> 1. Do you usually have a migraine or other headache more than two days per week?
> 2. Even though you use an acute migraine therapy, do you miss school, work, or family activities at least once per week because of your migraine?
> 3. Do you overuse acute migraine medications to prevent a migraine from occurring?
>
> If you answered "yes" to any of these questions, you should talk to your doctor about migraine prevention.

The simple, self-administered Migraine Prevention Quiz can be used by patients to determine if they may be candidates for preventive therapy (Box 6.1). Patient headache diaries should also be reviewed to determine actual headache frequency and medication use (see Chapter 4, Fig. 4.8). Preventive therapy, especially non-medication treatments, should be offered to all patients with frequent or disabling migraines.

> **Pearl for the practitioner:**
> Pregnant women who are likely to benefit from preventive medications can be identified by using the Migraine Preventive Quiz.

Provide Safe and Effective Prevention Recommendations

Effective preventive therapies include both non-medication and medication options. Women who may become or are already pregnant should receive extensive training in non-medication therapies, as outlined in Chapter 3. Preventive medications are typically reserved for those patients failing to achieve adequate headache control, despite good compliance with non-medication interventions. Patients requiring medication therapy should use drugs to complement rather than replace non-medication treatments. The combination of drug and non-drug approaches is usually more successful than either approach alone.

Consider Possible Future Pregnancy When Using Prevention in Non-pregnant Patients

When considering prescribing medications to any woman with childbearing potential, the clinician must always consider whether or not the patient is consistently using an effective form of contraception. This information should be reviewed at each visit. Unreliable use of effective contraception in sexually active patients or plans for conception in the near future should prompt the clinician to recommend those treatments that are known to be safe during conception and pregnancy.

> **Pearl for the practitioner:**
> When considering preventive medications in women who use unreliable methods of contraception or who are actively trying to get pregnant, the medications chosen should be considered safe if the woman were found to be pregnant.

Maximize Safe and Effective Non-medication Treatments

A wide variety of helpful non-medication treatments that can be used safely throughout preconception, pregnancy, and lactation are outlined in Chapter 3, with detailed patient instructions provided in Chapter 10 and on the accompanying CD. These therapies can be used by all headache patients and should be particularly encouraged in women of childbearing potential and those planning for pregnancy.

The most effective non-medication therapies include relaxation, with or without biofeedback, and stress management. Studies consistently show headache reduction from these therapies comparable to benefits achieved with prolonged use of standard headache prevention medications, like amitriptyline and propranolol. The good efficacy and excellent safety records with non-medications makes them ideal for women during conception, pregnancy, and lactation.

Benefits during pregnancy from minimal-therapist-contact relaxation techniques using thermal biofeedback plus neck exercises were demonstrated in a controlled clinical trial [2,3]. Pregnant women with problematic headaches were randomized to four treatment sessions learning thermal biofeedback plus neck exercises or to an attention control. The attention control group was provided with the same number of treatment sessions as the biofeedback group; however, they were not taught pain-reducing skills, but spent time discussing their headaches with the therapist. Headache activity was assessed in prospectively-recorded daily diaries before treatment and one month after completing treatment. Significant headache improvement (a reduction of $\geq 50\%$) occurred for

73% treated with biofeedback versus 29% assigned to the attention control [2]. Attention control patients were permitted to obtain active therapy after their post-treatment assessment, with no additional data collected. Headache activity was monitored throughout the remainder of pregnancy and up to one year postpartum for active treatment patients, with no additional treatment provided (Fig. 6.3). Benefits were maintained up to one year postpartum in 68% of treated subjects [3].

> **Pearl for the practitioner:**
> Relaxation methods, with or without biofeedback, and stress management are very effective non-drug options and should be utilized in all headache sufferers, especially those who are pregnant or may become pregnant.

Utilize Medications in Select, Difficult-to-treat Patients

Few drugs are FDA-approved as migraine preventive therapy (Box 6.2). Most preventive recommendations are based on clinical trials documenting benefit after drugs have been approved and available for treating other medical conditions, e.g., mood disorders, cardiovascular disease, and epilepsy. Most drugs have not been directly tested in clinical trials to determine safety for use during pregnancy, although FDA risk classifications are available to help guide medication selection (Box 6.3). While long-acting oxycodone is an FDA

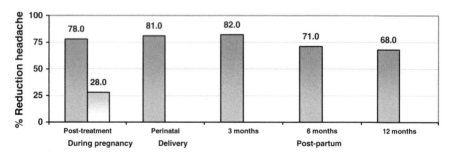

Fig. 6.3 Mean percentage reduction in headache activity after non-pharmacological treatment (Based on [2,3])
Post-treatment improvement was calculated one month after completing treatment. Headache activity was prospectively evaluated during the two weeks immediately before delivery (perinatal) and postpartum. Headache reduction of about 80% occurred with non-drug treatment, with good maintenance during pregnancy and through three months after delivery. A slight decline in reduction after three months suggests offering a training booster session six months after completing initial non-drug training sessions.

Box 6.2 FDA-approved drugs for migraine prevention in non-pregnant patients

- Methysergide maleate [Sansert—no longer available in the United States]
- Propranolol [Inderal]
- Timolol [Blocadren]
- Divalproex sodium [Depakote]
- Topiramate [Topamax]

Box 6.3 FDA risk classification of preventive headache medications during pregnancy and attempted conception

- FDA risk category B—safe
  - Long-acting oxycodone [Oxycontin]: long-acting opioids offer only modest benefit for chronic headache reduction and should only be used in highly selective, recalcitrant cases.

- FDA risk category C—use if benefit outweighs risk
  - Buproprion [Wellbutrin]
  - Gabapentin [Neurontin]
  - Lamotrigine [Lamictal]
  - Propranolol [Inderal]
  - Selective serotonin reuptake inhibitor antidepressants (except for paroxetine)
  - Timolol [Blocadren]
  - Topiramate [Topamax]
  - Tricyclic antidepressants
  - Venlafaxine [Effexor]
  - Verapamil [Calan, Isoptin, Verelan]

- FDA risk category D or X—avoid during pregnancy
  - Atenolol [Tenormin]
  - Divalproex sodium [Depakote]
  - Paroxetine [Paxil]

---

risk-category B drug, opioids offer minimal benefit for headache prevention and should generally be reserved for patients requiring specialist care for their headaches. Extensive testing of medication use in pregnant women is lacking. This limits the confidence that clinicians have in making recommendations about medication safety in pregnancy. Some medications, however, have been used more extensively in pregnant women, allowing for additional recommendations beyond simply relying on FDA risk categories.

Fortunately, data are available to help provide reasonable medication recommendations to pregnant patients with headaches. In some cases, the extensive use of preventive therapies to treat other, non-headache medical conditions provides helpful safety information. For example, safety data are available regarding the use of antihypertensives to treat pregnancy-related hypertension, antidepressants for mood disturbances, and antiepileptics for seizure disorders. In these cases, the risk of non-treatment of the disease often outweighs possible medication-effects, providing both anecdotal and large-scale experience in pregnant populations. European national registry databases also provide an excellent resource for collecting data on pregnancy outcome in women treated for chronic headache or other medical conditions, using various preventive therapies.

In addition to general medical databases, both disease- or medication-specific registries are available to log pregnancy outcome in women exposed to a variety of therapies during pregnancies [4]. In many cases, exposure may include only a single dose of a drug or limited duration of treatment in those patients inadvertently treated before pregnancy was identified. Obviously, data regarding single dose or limited duration exposure is less useful in making recommendations about long-term safety. In other cases where an underlying serious medical condition requires ongoing treatment, like depression or epilepsy, long-term exposure data are available. While most registries collect data for specific individual drugs or drug categories, the General Practice Research Database provides a computerized database of longitudinal medical records from primary care. Data are currently being collected on 3.4 million active patients from about 450 primary care practices in the United Kingdom. Information about contributing to the database and preliminary outcome data can be accessed at their website: http://www.gprd.com/home/ (Accessed March 2008). Data from these pregnancy-outcome collection systems will continue to provide updated information about the safety of medication exposures during pregnancy.

> **Pearl for the practitioner:**
> While data regarding use of preventive medications in pregnant women is not as robust as the data in non-pregnant patients, there is often enough information to make rational, safer recommendations for the minority of pregnant women who require them.

Don't Permit Analgesic Overuse in Patients Needing Prevention

Patients and their healthcare providers are often more comfortable with the use of over-the-counter analgesic medications rather than prescription therapy. A longitudinal study of 2,086 women attending one of four rural obstetric clinics

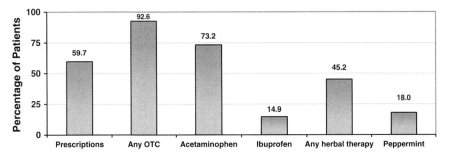

Fig. 6.4 Percentage of patients using medications during pregnancy (Based on [5])
Prescriptions category excludes prenatal vitamins and iron. OTC = over-the-counter drug.

revealed that almost all of the women used over-the-counter medications, most commonly acetaminophen (Fig. 6.4) [5]. Herbal remedies were used by almost as many as those using prescription medications, most commonly peppermint. These data highlight the predominant widespread use of non-prescription drugs during pregnancy, especially analgesics. Failure to adequately assess headache and medication use patterns may result in the overuse of over-the-counter analgesics. Excessive use of analgesics may result in both medication-related side effects and headache aggravation with the development of analgesic overuse headaches. Medication overuse can be identified and minimized by routine dialogues about both prescription and non-prescription treatment use at each office visit.

> ***Pearl for the practitioner:***
> Clinicians should routinely ask pregnant women about their use of prescription and non-prescription medication for pain and other symptoms—both those prescribed by other providers and over-the-counter remedies. Don't assume that women are not taking medications during pregnancy.

The negative impact from overusing analgesics or other acute headache therapies is highlighted by studies documenting headache reduction from discontinuation of excessive acute treatment. In one study, fifty patients with chronic migraine and daily or near daily headache for at least six months were required to discontinue all overused acute treatment, with no additional therapy for the first week. At baseline, all patients reported moderate (26%) or more severe headaches (74%). One week after discontinuing medications, 25% of patients reported no headache, 23% mild headache, 24% moderate headache, and 28% severe headache [6]. After one week, patients with headache were treated with preventive therapy, with further improvement likely due to the combination of both medication withdrawal and appropriate prevention care. In another study, patients overusing analgesics were treated with analgesic detoxification and followed for two months [7]. The average reduction in the number of days with headache was 68% following analgesic detoxification. Interestingly, patients treated with detoxification alone experienced a similar outcome to those treated with detoxification plus additional preventive therapy and prednisone. These data emphasize the central role that medication withdrawal plays in reducing headaches in patients experiencing medication overuse headaches.

Recommendations are sometimes made for patients to consider daily, low-dose analgesic therapy as headache prevention. This is problematic because the development of medication overuse headache is more related to the number of days when medication is taken than to the doses taken per day. In general, regularly using analgesics three or more days per week results in a substantial risk for the development of analgesic overuse headaches. Patients using low-dose, cardioprotective aspirin, however, generally do not experience headache aggravation. Nevertheless, low-dose aspirin has not been shown to produce significant decreases in migraine activity and should not be recommended as headache prevention treatment [8].

> **Pearl for the practitioner:**
> All analgesic medication (including prescribed and over-the-counter drugs) should be limited to two days per week or less on a regular basis to avoid developing analgesic rebound headache.

Limit Preventive Medication Exposure

When a woman experiences frequent headaches during her pregnancy, she should be informed that headaches often improve after the first trimester. Non-drug treatment options should always be considered initially. These options were discussed in detail in Chapter 3 and include sleep and meal regulation, trigger identification and avoidance, cognitive behavioral therapy, relaxation, biofeedback, physical therapy, and massage therapy. These are particularly important in the first trimester, when organogenesis occurs and medication is best avoided if possible.

When headaches persist into the second and third trimester or are particularly frequent and/or severe later in the first trimester, preventive medication can be considered. It is imperative that the headache-treating physician work closely with the obstetrician if preventive medications are to be used. It is preferable to use safer, effective preventive medications in appropriate patients rather than allowing the patient to overuse analgesic medications. Brief descriptions of each of the major classes of preventive medications are provided below.

Pearl for the practitioner:
It is preferable to use a safer preventive medication in pregnant women than to allow them to overuse analgesic medications.

Antihypertensives

Among headache preventive medications, beta-blockers have the best track record for a combination of good efficacy and safety in pregnant women. Due to widespread use for safely managing hypertension during pregnancy, propranolol [Inderal] is usually considered to be first-line therapy for women requiring a medication preventive for chronic headaches. Beta-blocker exposure may, however, increase the risk for neonatal hypoglycemia, hypotension, bradycardia, and respiratory depression. They should also be used with caution in women who have asthma, baseline low blood pressure, or baseline bradycardia. Atenolol [Tenormin] exposure at conception or during the first trimester has been linked to low birth weight [9]. Older studies have similarly suggested a possible association between propranolol and intrauterine growth retardation. Ideally, beta-blockers should be tapered within the last few weeks of pregnancy (starting around week 36) to minimize effects on labor and the newborn baby.

Other hypertensives have also shown moderate efficacy as headache preventives, including calcium channel blockers, the angiotensin converting enzyme inhibitor lisinopril, and the angiotensin II receptor antagonist candesartan. Calcium channel blockers are the best studied non-beta blocker group, with flunarizine [not available in the United States] the most effective of this group. The calcium channel blocker verapamil [Calan, Isoptin, Verelan] is listed as an FDA risk category C medication. While calcium channel blockers were not linked to increased risk of malformations in a large, Hungarian surveillance survey, experience in pregnancy is inadequate to recommend routine use for headache prevention during pregnancy [10]. Furthermore, efficacy as headache prevention in non-pregnant patients is generally less with calcium channel blockers than with beta blockers. Lisinopril has been linked to teratogenicity and toxicity in the fetus and newborn after the first trimester and should be avoided [11]. Candesartan has less literature available describing its use during pregnancy; however, its similarity in mechanism to lisinopril suggests avoiding candesartan as a headache prevention therapy in these patients.

Pearl for the practitioner:
If antihypertensive medications are being considered for headache prevention during pregnancy, propranolol is preferred due to extensive clinical experience.

Antiepileptics

Although antiepileptic medications can effectively prevent migraine, their use is typically restricted during pregnancy. Divalproex sodium (valproate plus valproic acid [Depakote]), is absolutely contraindicated during conception and pregnancy, due to teratogenic effects with neural tube defects and reduced clotting in the mother and baby. Gabapentin [Neurontin] is a moderately effective migraine preventive therapy, although clinical trials have not directly assessed its use in pregnant migraineurs [12]. Gabapentin is an FDA pregnancy risk category C drug and is typically discontinued in the 3rd trimester because of possible interference with bony development. Small studies in epileptic women have not identified fetal effects with gabapentin treatment [13]. The Gabapentin Pregnancy Registry published data on 44 live births, with no increased risk of abortion, low birth weight, or malformation seen in gabapentin-exposed babies [13]. The very small number in this sample, however, substantially limits safety interpretations that can be made using these data. Data on patients exposed to gabapentin may be entered into this registry by calling 617-638-7751. Although efficacy is superior with topiramate [Topamax], limited clinical experience and early malformation reports suggest restricting topiramate use as a migraine preventive during pregnancy. Post-marketing data reported topiramate exposure in male babies with hypospadia [14]. A single case report described the occurrence of limb and oral malformations in offspring of a woman treated for epilepsy during pregnancy with topiramate [15]. Furthermore, preliminary data from the prospective UK Epilepsy and Pregnancy Register catalogued congenital malformations associated with first trimester exposure to topiramate, which included two cases of cleft lip and palate and one of hypospadias in the offspring of 70 women using topiramate monotherapy [16]. Five minor malformations were also reported: sacral dimple, clicky hips, plagiocephaly (an asymmetrical skull deformity from irregular closure of the cranial sutures), toe webbing, and immature hip joints. Thus, topiramate cannot be recommended at this time as a safe headache preventive medication option in pregnancy.

The International Registry of Antiepileptic Drugs and Pregnancy (EURAP) has collected data from Europe, Australia, Asia, and South America. An interim report in November of 2007 included data for 4,833 prospective pregnancies (available at http://www.eurapinternational.org; accessed July 2008). There were 277 major malformations and 43 chromosomal/monogenic abnormalities. Among patients treated with antiepileptic monotherapy, birth defects occurred in 6.5%. The large North American Antiepileptic Drug Pregnancy Registry sponsored by Massachusetts General Hospital (http://www.massgeneral.org/aed/; accessed July 2008) is collecting data on the outcome of intrauterine exposure to antiepileptic drugs for treating seizures or other medical conditions (like migraine prevention). Patients may be enrolled by calling 888-233-2334. As with the European registry, six-year experience data reported major malformation in 6.5% with monotherapy phenobarbital exposure [17]. Publication of 10-year data is planned for 2009. Preliminary 10-year data revealed a clear association with maternal monotherapy with phenopbarbital or valproate with congenital malformations [18]. Over 900 infants had been exposed to monotherapy with either carbamazepine or lamotrigine, with identification of an increased risk for the occurrence of cleft palate [19]. Exposure to monotherapy with other drugs was insufficient at the time of this report to determine reliable risks, as 500–600 exposed infants are probably needed before risk determination becomes valid.

> **Pearl for the practitioner:**
> Although antiepileptic drugs are among the most effective preventive agents for migraine, their use in pregnancy is limited. Depakote should be avoided. Topiramate has insufficient available data to permit safe recommendation. Gabapentin (FDA risk category C), though possibly less effective, is the safest of the three agents and may be used in early pregnancy.

Antidepressants

Antidepressants, especially tricyclics, are among the most effective prevention medications in non-pregnant patients; however, they should be limited during pregnancy. A recent meta-analysis evaluated studies reporting rates of spontaneous abortion in women using antidepressants ($N = 1,534$) compared with non-depressed women ($N = 2,033$) [20]. The rate of spontaneous abortion was higher in the depressed women treated with antidepressants (12% vs. 4%, relative risk $= 1.45$). No differences were found among antidepressant classes. Although these data do not determine whether the increased miscarriage rate was due to depression-related factors or to medication use, antidepressants should probably be selected after first considering and/or failing beta-blockers and gabapentin in pregnant women.

Tricyclic antidepressants are the most effective class of mood stabilizers for headache prevention. Tricyclics are FDA risk category C, with early reports suggesting a link with cardiac and limb malformations. Selective serotonin reuptake inhibitors (SSRIs) are sometimes used as second-line treatment in non-pregnant patients, although SSRIs are substantially less effective for headache prevention than tricyclic antidepressants. Exposure to SSRIs during pregnancy has been linked to increased risk for low birth weight and respiratory distress [21]. Most SSRI antidepressants are listed as FDA risk category C; however, paroxetine [Paxil] was recently reassigned to category D, after identification of an increased risk of congenital heart defects. Recently, paroxetine exposure during the first trimester was associated with an increased risk of major malformations (odds ratio = 2.2) and major cardiac malformations (odds ratio = 3.1) only among women using a daily dosage >25 mg [22]. Third trimester treatment with either tricyclic or SSRI antidepressants has been linked to increased perinatal complications, including respiratory distress, endocrine and metabolic disorders, and temperature regulation disturbances [23].

Furthermore, the use of serotonin reuptake inhibitors, including SSRIs and serotonin and norepinephrine reuptake inhibitors, in the third trimester has been linked to a behavioral neonatal syndrome [24]. In comparison to babies with no in utero exposure to serotonin reuptake inhibitors or exposure during early pregnancy, babies exposed in the third trimester carry a risk ratio of 3.0 for the development of neonatal behavioral syndrome. Most cases have been reported with fluoxetine [Prozac] and paroxetine. Features typically include tremors/jitteriness, increased muscle tone/reflexes, feeding/digestive disturbances, irritability/agitation, respiratory disturbances, excessive crying, and sleep disturbances. In most cases, symptoms are mild and respond to supportive measures.

Bupropion [Wellbutrin], another antidepressant with some benefit for headache prevention, is also an FDA pregnancy risk category C drug [25,26]. Pregnancy registry data identified a higher than expected incidence of cardiac abnormalities in babies exposed to bupropion in utero [27]. A small, prospective study compared pregnancy outcome in 136 women using bupropion at least during their first trimester and in 133 controls [28]. Bupropion was used throughout pregnancy in 45 of these women. Malformations were similar between the two groups; however, bupropion-exposed women experienced a significantly higher rate of spontaneous abortion (15% vs. 4%, $P = 0.009$). A recent review of data from 1,213 infants exposed to bupropion during the first trimester showed no increased malformation risk compared with infants using other antidepressants ($N = 4,743$) or bupropion outside of the first trimester ($N = 1,049$) [29].

> **Pearl for the practitioner:**
> While antidepressants may be necessary to treat severe mood disorders during pregnancy, they are infrequently recommended as headache prevention during pregnancy, due to small risks identified with most groups of antidepressants in both early and late pregnancy.

Injections and Alternative Therapies

In uncontrolled studies, peripheral nerve injections, most commonly occipital nerve blocks and trigger point injections, may reduce headache activity in patients with frequent, recalcitrant headaches [30,31].

Anatomic studies show that the greater occipital nerve can be located 22% of the distance between the external occipital protuberance and the mastoid process (Fig. 6.5) [32]. The nerve is, therefore, typically located about 2 cm lateral to the external occipital protuberance [32]. Autopsy studies have shown a significant degree of anatomic variation among individuals regarding the exact location of the greater and lesser occipital nerves . This argues for a wider than usual distribution of medication to effectively block both the greater and lesser occipital nerves. In one series, 46% of unilateral greater occipital nerve blocks administered to migraine patients resulted in complete or partial pain relief [33]. Each block used a 3 mL mixture of 2% lidocaine and 80 mg of methylprednisolone. Most patients experienced complete relief for seven days, with a mean duration of relief of 20 days. Partial response lasted for 20 days in most patients, with a mean duration of partial response of 45 days. Pretreatment tenderness over the greater occipital nerve predicted success. Patients with head pain originating from the base of the skull or top of the neck and radiating over the head, as well as those patients with tenderness over the occipital nerve, may benefit from a trial with occipital nerve blocks. These procedures are safe and effective and can be learned by interested providers. Other blocks, such as C2 nerve blocks

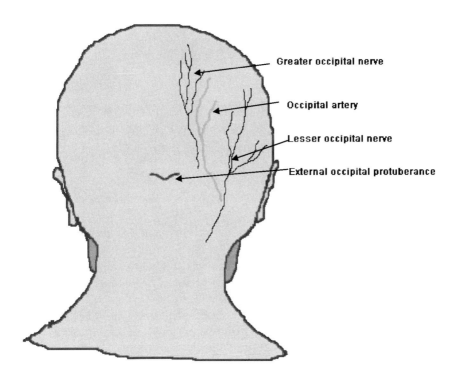

Fig. 6.5 Occipital nerve anatomy

and cervical facet blocks, though usually done by interventional pain specialists, can also be useful with minimal side effects. There is a paucity of data regarding these interventional pain procedures in pregnant women.

Botulinum toxin type A is routinely used in cosmetic procedures to reduce facial lines and has been tested in multiple trials as a migraine preventive agent. A recent review evaluating the published efficacy of migraine preventive therapies determined that the available evidence does not support recommending botulinum toxin injections as an effective migraine prevention therapy [34]. Therefore, botulinum toxin injections should not be offered to either pregnant or non-pregnant migraine sufferers. For those women who have used botulinum toxin during pregnancy, a recent report described two women who were inadvertently administered botulinum toxin injections for cosmetic indications during the early first trimester before either woman was aware that she was pregnant [35]. Healthy, term babies were delivered in both cases. While experience in only two women is not adequate to support safe use, these data may offer comfort to patients who have also been inadvertently exposed. Other muscle relaxant therapies similarly have a limited role in headache prevention in non-pregnant patients and have not established robust safety records during pregnancy.

Acupuncture has also been tested as a migraine preventive therapy. Studies consistently show no better result from patients randomized to receive real acupuncture versus sham acupuncture [34]. Therefore, acupuncture should not be offered to either non-pregnant or pregnant migraine patients.

> **Pearl for the practitioner:**
> Occipital nerve blocks may effectively relieve headaches. Neither botulinum toxin nor acupuncture has demonstrated reliable benefit for headache relief.

Vitamins, Herbs, and Supplements

A variety of vitamins, minerals, herbs, and other supplements can effectively reduce primary headaches, especially migraine in non-pregnant women; these include feverfew, butterbur, and coenzyme Q10. Due to lack of safety data, these therapies should *not* be used during pregnancy. Magnesium and high-dose riboflavin may also reduce migraines in non-pregnant patients, although consistent benefits with riboflavin have not been demonstrated in such patients. Furthermore, the safety of high-dose riboflavin has not been established during pregnancy. Recent recommendations from the European Federation of Neurological Societies based on review of scientific data from clinical trials and expert consensus opinion support using magnesium as a headache preventive during pregnancy [36].

Ginseng is also sometimes used for migraine prevention. Analysis of data from a pregnancy cohort study in which 0.8% of women used ginseng during the first trimester of pregnancy found no increased malformation risk linked to ginseng use [37]. Because of a paucity of data demonstrating efficacy, ginseng is generally not recommended.

> ***Pearl for the practitioner:***
> Among nutritional/supplement treatments, only magnesium is recommended as a headache preventive during pregnancy.

Summarizing Medication Recommendations

In general, preventive treatment should be offered to patients continuing to report headaches at the end of their first trimester. Initial treatment selection should focus on effective non-medication therapies, like relaxation and biofeedback, that produce comparable efficacy to standard medications and have directly demonstrated benefit in pregnant headache sufferers. Patients requiring medication therapy should limit treatment to medications with the best safety records, including propranolol, gabapentin in early pregnancy, and magnesium (Table 6.1).

Table 6.1 Prevention medication recommendations during pregnancy

Drug	FDA Class	Dose	Comments
Magnesium oxide	Not rated	200–300 mg BID or 400 mg once daily	May cause diarrhea or stomach upset.
Propranolol [Inderal]	C	40–240 mg daily. Available as short-acting or extended-release preparations.	Taper after week 36. Monitor baby for bradycardia, hypoglycemia, and respiratory distress. Extensive clinical experience during pregnancy. Avoid in women with low blood pressure, bradycardia, or asthma
Gabapentin [Neurontin]	C	100–600 mg TID	Use only during conception and early pregnancy. Discontinue in third trimester.

BID = two times daily, TID = three times daily

Summary

While most pregnant women with headaches note significant improvement in their headache pattern after the first trimester, a substantial minority do not. This group can be identified by using the Migraine Preventive Quiz. For those patients likely to have persistent severe headaches throughout their pregnancy, preventive treatment options should be considered. It is far better to use a safe preventive agent than allow the pregnant women to overuse analgesic medications, hoping that the headache pattern will spontaneously improve.

Practical pointers:

- Non-drug treatment options, especially stress management and relaxation techniques with or without biofeedback, should be offered to all pregnant women, particularly those with disabling headaches.
- Preventive medications should be considered for patients with frequent, severe, disabling headaches not responding to non-drug therapies.
- Only those medications considered safe in early pregnancy should be prescribed to fertile women using unreliable methods of contraception or who are actively trying to get pregnant.
- Medications should be limited during pregnancy, if possible. If preventive medications are used, those with the best safety and efficacy data should be used, e.g., propranlolol, gabapentin (in early pregnancy), and magnesium.
- Failure to provide effective prevention therapy may result in unnecessary disability and the overuse of acute headache medications.

References

1. Marcus DA, Scharff L, Turk DC. Longitudinal prospective study of headache during pregnancy and postpartum. *Headache* 1999;39:625–632.
2. Marcus DA, Scharff L, Turk DC. Nonpharmacologial management of headaches during pregnancy. *Psychosom Med* 1995;57:527–535.
3. Scharff L, Marcus DA, Turk DC. Maintenance of effects in the nonmedical treatment of headaches during pregnancy. *Headache* 1996;36:285–290.
4. Charlton RA, Cunnington MC, de Vries CS, Weil JG. Data resources for investigating drug exposure during pregnancy and associated outcomes. The General Practice Research Database (GPRD) as an alternative to pregnancy registries. *Drug Saf* 2008;31:39–51.
5. Glover DD, Amonkar M, Rybeck BF, Tracy TS. Prescription, over-the-counter, and herbal medicine use in a rural, obstetric population. *Am J Obstet Gynecol* 2003;188:1039–1045.
6. Krymchantowski AV, Moreira PF. Out-patient detoxification in chronic migraine: comparison of strategies. *Cephalalgia* 2003;23:982–993.

7. Rossi P, Di Lorenzo C, Faroni J, Cesarion F, Nappi G. Advice alone vs. structured detoxification programmes for medication overuse headaches: a prospective, randomized, open-label trial in transformed migraine patients with low medical needs. *Cephalalgia* 2006;26:1097–1105.

8. Benseñor IM, Cook NR, Lee IM, et al. Low-dose aspirin for migraine prophylaxis in women. *Cephalalgia* 2001;21:175–183.

9. Bayliss H, Churchill D, Beevers M, Beevers DG. Anti-hypertensive drugs in pregnancy and fetal growth: evidence for "pharmacological programming" in the first trimester? *Hypertens Pregnancy* 2002;21:161–174.

10. Sørensen HT, Czeizel AE, Rockerbauer M, Steffensen FH, Olsen J. The risk of limb deficiencies and other congenital malformations in children exposed in utero to calcium channel blockers. *Acta Obstet Gynecol Scand* 2001;80:397–401.

11. Drug Safety Site.com: http://drugsafetysite.com/lisinopril (accessed June 2008).

12. Mathew NT, Rapoport A, Saper J, et al. Efficacy of gabapentin in migraine prophylaxis. *Headache* 2001;41:119–128.

13. Montouris G. Gabapentin exposure in human pregnancy: results from the Gabapentin Pregnancy Registry. *Epilepsy Behav* 2003;4:310–317.

14. Topiramate (TOPAMAX) prescribing information. In: Physicians' Desk Reference 2007. Montvale, NJ: Thomson Healthcare;2007;2408.

15. Vila Cerén C, Demestre Guasch X, Raspall Torrent F, et al. Topiramate and pregnancy. Neonate with bone anomalies. *An Pediatr (Barc)* 2005;63:363–365.

16. Hunt S, Russell A, Smithson WH, et al. Topiramate in pregnancy: preliminary experience from the UK Epilepsy and Pregnancy Register. *Neurology* 2008; 71:272–276.

17. Holmes LB, Wyszynski DF, Lieberman E. The AED (Antiepileptic Drug) pregnancy registry. *Arch Neurol* 2004;61:673–678.

18. Holmes LB, Smith CR, Hernandez-Diaz S. Pregnancy registries: larger sample sizes essential. *Birth Defects Research (Part A)* 2008;82:307.

19. Holmes LB, Baldwin EJ, Smith CR, Habecker E, Glassman L, Wong SL, Wyszynski DF. Increased frequency of isolated cleft palate in infants exposed to lamotrigine during pregnancy. *Neurology* 2008;70:2152–2158.

20. Hemels ME, Einarson A, Koren G, Lanctot KL, Einarson TR. Antidepressant use during pregnancy and the rates of spontaneous abortions: a meta-analysis. *Ann Pharmacother* 2005;39:803–809.

21. Oberlander TF, Warburton W, Misri A, Aghajanian J, Hertzman C. Neonatal outcomes after prenatal exposure to selective serotonin reuptake inhibitor antidepressants and maternal depression using population-based linked health data. *Arch Gen Psychiatry* 2006;63:898–906.

22. Bérard A, Ramos E, Rey E, et al. First trimester exposure to paroxetine and risk of cardiac malformations in infants: the importance of dosage. *Birth Defects Res B Dev Reprod Toxicol* 2007;80:18–27.

23. Davis RL, Rubanowice D, McPhillips H, et al. Risks of congenital malformations and perinatal events among infants exposed to antidepressant medications during pregnancy. *Pharmacoepidemiol Drug Saf* 2007;16:1086–1094.

24. Moses-Kolko EL, Bogen D, Perel J, et al. Neonatal signs after late in utero exposure to serotonin reuptake inhibitors: literature review and implications for clinical applications. *JAMA* 2005;293:2372–2383.

25. Goodman JF: Treatment of headache with bupropion. *Headache* 1997;37:256.

26. Pinsker W: Potentially safe and effective new treatment for migraine? *Headache* 1998;38:58.

27. No authors. Bupropion (amfebutamone): caution during pregnancy. *Prescrire Int* 2005;14:225.

28. Chun-Fai-Chan B, Koren G, Fayez I, et al. Pregnancy outcome of women exposed to bupropion during pregnancy: a prospective comparative study. *Am J Obstet Gynecol* 2005;192:932–936.
29. Cole JA, Modell JG, Haight BR, et al. Bupropion in pregnancy and the prevalence of congenital malformations. *Pharmacoepidemiol Drug Saf* 2007;16:474–484.
30. Ashkenazi A, Levin M. Greater occipital nerve block for migraine and other headaches: is it useful? *Curr Pain Headache Rep* 2007;11:231–235.
31. Ashkenazi AA, Matro R, Shaw JW, Abbas MA, Silberstein SD. Greater occipital nerve block using local anesthestics alone or with triamcinolone for transformed migraine: a randomized comparative study. *J Neurol Neurosurg Psychiatry* 2008;79:415–417.
32. Loukas M, El-Sedfy A, Tubbs RS, et al. Identification of greater occipital nerve landmarks for the treatment of occipital neuralgia. *Folia Morph* 2006;65:337–342.
33. Afridi SK, Shields KG, Bhola R, Goadsby PJ. Greater occipital nerve injection in primary headache symptoms—prolonged effects from a single injection. *Pain* 2006;122:126–129.
34. Schürks M, Diener H, Goadsby P. Update on the prophylaxis of migraine. *Curr Treat Opt Neurol* 2008;10:20–29.
35. De Oliveira Monteiro E. Botulinum toxin and pregnancy. *Skinmed* 2006;5:308.
36. Evers S, Áfra J, Frese A, et al. EFNS guideline on the drug treatment of migraine—report of an EFNS task force. *Eur J Neurol* 2006;13:560–572.
37. Chuang C, Doyle P, Wang J, et al. Herbal medicines used during the first trimester and major congenital malformations. An analysis of data from a pregnancy cohort study. *Drug Saf* 2006;29:537–548.

Chapter 7
Preventive Treatment Options for the Lactating Headache Patient

Key Chapter Points

- Headache sufferers should be informed that chronic headaches typically recur postpartum, even for patients who became headache-free during pregnancy.
- Fatigue, lack of sleep, significant changes in routine, and dropping estrogen levels all combine to lower the headache threshold after delivery.
- A plan for preventive therapy should be developed before delivery for patients who needed preventive therapy prior to pregnancy.
- Late pregnancy provides an ideal opportunity for non-medication therapy training, in preparation for headache return postpartum.
- Preferred preventive headache medications for lactating women are propranolol and timolol. Verapamil may also be used, although headache efficacy is less. Divalproex sodium, while contraindicated during pregnancy, may be safely used postpartum in patients with reliable contraception.
- Magnesium may be offered to patients preferring nutritional prevention.

Keywords American Academy of Pediatrics · Breastfeeding · Nursing · Postpartum

> *I felt so great during my pregnancy. I had morning sickness and back aches, but my migraines were completely gone! It was wonderful! When I saw my obstetrician for my first postpartum visit, I was only getting infrequent, minor headaches, so I didn't say anything. For the last two months, my migraines have been as bad as they were before my pregnancy. I couldn't get an appointment to see my doctor for several weeks, so I figured I'd better quit breastfeeding so I could go back on my Inderal, which worked so well before. I had an old prescription I've been taking and my headaches are finally under good control again. I do feel guilty about not nursing Emma very long—but what else could I have done?*

Women are often surprised about and unprepared for the usually inevitable return of chronic headaches after delivery. Inadequate preparation prior to

D.A. Marcus, P.A. Bain, *Effective Migraine Treatment in Pregnant and Lactating Women: A Practical Guide*, DOI 10.1007/978-1-60327-439-5_7, © Humana Press, a part of Springer Science+Business Media, LLC 2009

delivery can unfortunately result in unnecessary pain, disability, and, as described by our patient above, needless stopping or avoiding of breastfeeding. The healthcare provider and patient should develop plans for headache treatment after delivery, when headaches are likely to recur. This chapter will review treatment options for nursing women whose headaches are frequent and/or severe enough to warrant preventive therapy.

A number of reasons, including the need to use medications, impact decisions to discontinue nursing prematurely. Over 1,000 low-risk mothers were followed prospectively after delivery to gather information about breastfeeding habits [1]. A total of 87% of the women were breastfeeding 1–2 days after delivery, 75% after 2 weeks, and 55% after 12 weeks. The most common reason for discontinuing breastfeeding during the first 3 postpartum weeks was a perception that the baby was not receiving enough milk (Table 7.1). The mother becoming ill or needing to take a medication was reported as the reason for

Table 7.1 Most common reasons for prematurely discontinuing breastfeeding (Based on [1])

Reason for discontinuation	Percentage citing specific reason
Birth to postpartum week 1	
Infant still hungry/insufficient milk	27
Problems with latching on/sucking	23
Other*	18
Breast pain	14
Convenience of bottle feeding	8
Return to school/work	4
Lack of energy/desire to breastfeed	4
Mother sick or on medication	2
Postpartum weeks 2–3	
Infant still hungry/insufficient milk	18
Breast pain	14
Return to school/work	14
Other*	13
Mother sick or on medication	12
Problems with latching on/sucking	12
Convenience of bottle feeding	9
Lack of energy/desire to breastfeed	8
Postpartum weeks 10–12	
Return to school/work	58
Mother sick or on medication	11
Infant still hungry/insufficient milk	11
Other*	11
Problems with latching on/sucking	5
Lack of energy/desire to breastfeed	4

*Other includes infant not gaining weight or sick, breast milk intolerance, and spitting up.

discontinuing nursing by >10% of women after the second postpartum week. After 10 weeks, the only reason more often given for discontinuation of breast-feeding than maternal illness or medication use was returning to school or work. While this study did not specify individual illnesses that were being treated in these women, healthcare providers should be aware that there are many rela-tively safe and effective treatment options for disabling headaches that can allow the postpartum headache sufferer to continue nursing.

> ***Pearl for the practitioner:***
> Postpartum headaches can be disabling for women and result in unneces-sary discontinuation of breastfeeding. Many safer treatment options are available that can effectively reduce headache-related disability and allow the woman to continue nursing.

Plan for Headache Recurrence After Delivery

As described in Chapter 5, although headache recurrence is delayed with breastfeeding, migraine recurrence affects one in five women one week after delivery and two in five women after one month [2]. Plans for headache prevention should be formulated prior to delivery, especially for women who experienced frequent headaches before pregnancy.

Include Plans for Contraception

Contraception after delivery can be achieved with condoms, spermicides, and/ or an intrauterine device. Combined hormonal contraceptives are not recom-mended during the immediate postpartum period, while progestin-only pre-parations may be used. Furthermore, estrogen is associated with reduced milk production [3]. Patients interested in resuming certain antiepileptic drugs post-partum should be cautioned about possible oral contraceptive failure and unintended pregnancy. Several antiepileptic drugs, including topiramate, induce the hepatic cytochrome P450 3A4 enzyme system [4]. Concomitant use with oral contraceptives, therefore, may result in failure of oral contraceptives. This potential interaction does not occur with valproate or gabapentin. For-tunately, serum estrogen concentrations from oral contraceptives are not expected to be reduced until topiramate concentrations reach 200 mg daily or higher and typical dosages for migraine prevention are 50 mg twice daily or less [5]. Patients interested in resuming divalproex sodium need to verify consistent use of reliable contraception to minimize the risk for inadvertent pregnancy.

Pearl for the practitioner:
Women who are taking topiramate and an estrogen-containing OCP do not have to be concerned about decreased effectiveness of the OCP until the topiramate daily dose exceeds 200 mg (higher than usually required for effective headache treatment).

Pearl for the practitioner:
Verify reliable contraception before prescribing after delivery. Reliable postpartum contraception must be ensured before prescribing drugs with potentially teratogenic effects, such as valproate.

Develop a Safe and Effective Preventive Treatment Plan

Maximize Effective Non-medication Treatments

Patients should be offered training and treatment with effective, non-medication options (see Chapter 3 for details). Training can be effectively achieved in the headache-free patient in preparation for later return of headaches, similar to instruction in Lamaze techniques in the months prior to delivery. Skills such as relaxation with or without biofeedback have demonstrated efficacy for headache prevention postpartum and in nursing mothers in controlled trials [6,7]. Although benefits from pain management training continue long-term, efficacy has been shown to dampen several months after initial training. Therefore, women who have been previously instructed in non-medication treatments may benefit from brief retraining during their final trimester of pregnancy, so they are confident in using skills when headaches return after delivery. Training during a period of headache quiescence can maximize patient focus on skill acquisition.

Select Safe Medications

In 2001, the American Academy of Pediatrics published a listing of medications considered to be compatible with breastfeeding [8]. Both the American Academy of Pediatrics (http://aappolicy.aappublications.org/) and the World Health Organization (http://www.who.int/child-adolescent-health/) provide online resources cataloguing drug safety. Additional information about drug use during lactation can be found online at the Drugs and Lactation Database (LactMed at http://toxnet.nlm.nih.gov/), managed by the United States

National Library of Medicine. Information may also be obtained from a website managed by Thomas W. Hale, RPh, PhD, Professor of Pediatrics at Texas Tech University (http://neonatal.ttuhsc.edu/lact/). The latter site features an online forum with the option for healthcare providers to ask questions about specific medications not already listed.

Several compounds are considered relatively safe in nursing mothers (Box 7.1). As discussed in Chapter 2, various factors are important in determining how much medication gets passed from the mother to the infant via breast milk. Drug safety may depend on the age of the nursing baby, with the capacity to absorb and eliminate drugs being different in premature infants and newborns relative to older babies. In general, extra caution should be exercised when administering drugs to nursing mothers of premature babies or infants <1 month old. The following sections summarize the safety and efficacy of various preventive agents, grouped by class.

Box 7.1 Headache prevention drugs considered to be compatible with breastfeeding (Based on [8])

- Divalporex sodium [Depakote] (if using adequate contraception)
- Magnesium
- Propranolol [Inderal]
- Timolol [Blocadren]
- Verapamil [Calan]

Antihypertensives

Maternal use of the beta-blockers propranolol, timolol, and naldolol is considered to be compatible with breastfeeding, although the baby should be monitored for possible cardiovascular and respiratory effects (e.g., bradycardia, hypotension, and decreased or labored respiratory status) [8]. The American Academy of Pediatrics considers atenolol to be compatible with breastfeeding if caution is used, while the World Health Organization classification recommends avoiding atenolol. The relative infant dose with atenolol (7–19%) is substantially higher than with propranolol (0.2%), similarly favoring propranolol [9]. Therefore, propranolol and timolol are preferred therapies as they are both FDA-approved for migraine and are considered compatible with breastfeeding. Beta-blockers should not be used in women with a history of reactive airway disease (e.g., asthma). Verapamil is also compatible with breastfeeding, although headache relief is generally more effective with beta-blockers. Both propranolol and verapamil are available as sustained-release products, allowing once daily dosing to minimize the baby's exposure. Lack of available data prohibits offering safety recommendations for lisinopril or candesartan. Similar agents, enalapril and captopril, are listed as compatible with breastfeeding, although they have not been studied as headache preventives [8]. Superior efficacy and stronger safety information for propranolol and timolol suggests favoring these treatments if antihypertensives will be offered while nursing.

> **Pearl for the practitioner:**
> Propranolol and timolol are compatible with nursing and are the preferred antihypertensive agents for headache prevention.

Antiepileptics

Divalproex sodium [Depakote] is compatible with breastfeeding in women consistently using effective contraception [8]. The amount of valproic acid transferring to the infant via milk is low. Breastfeeding is safe, although like the mother, the infant needs monitoring of liver and platelet activity. Women taking divalproex sodium should be regularly questioned about contraceptive use to ensure safe continuation with a low risk of inadvertent pregnancy. They should also be supplemented with folate.

> **Pearl for the practitioner:**
> Valproate is compatible with breastfeeding when adequate contraception is guaranteed to avoid inadvertent exposure of an unplanned pregnancy to this teratogen.

Other antiepileptics are generally not recommended as headache prevention while nursing, because of lack of available data to formulate rational safety recommendations. Topiramate [Topamax] is excreted into breast milk; however, limited data are available to determine possible effects of maternal topiramate on the nursing baby. Therefore, topiramate is generally avoided while nursing. Similarly, the transfer of gabapentin to breast milk is substantial; however, plasma concentrations in nursing infants are low, with no adverse effects reported in exposed infants in the literature [10,11]. Despite lack of reports of negative effects, gabapentin is also not recommended with nursing because headache prevention benefits are typically less than with other prevention therapies that have more robust safety records, such as propranolol.

Antidepressants

The American Academy of Pediatrics notes that maternal antidepressants have not been linked to specific effects in the baby, with the exception of fluoxetine, which can cause colic, irritability, feeding and sleep disorders, and slow weight gain [8]. Antidepressants, however, are of potential concern because they are excreted in breast milk and the effects on the baby's developing nervous system are unknown. Consequently, use of antidepressants as headache preventive therapy should be limited to patients failing treatments with more established safety records, such as propranolol and timolol. The Academy of Breastfeeding Medicine Protocol Committee recently published guidelines governing the use of antidepressants in nursing mothers [12]. Antidepressants were recommended only for women with moderate-to-severe depressive symptoms. While tricyclics and serotonin reuptake inhibitors were considered to be relatively safe, they suggested considering sertraline as first-line antidepressant therapy, due to lower levels in breast milk and infant serum. Other antidepressants might be considered first-line in those women with depression who had previously responded to an alternative therapy. Sertraline is much less effective as a headache prevention therapy than tricyclic antidepressants.

> *Pearl for the practitioner:*
> Antidepressants are typically restricted during nursing to the treatment of moderate-to-severe depression rather than used for headache prevention. Tricyclics and sertraline may be considered as second-line therapy in patients failing to achieve adequate headache control with beta-blockers and non-drug treatments.

Muscle Relaxants

In general, muscle relaxants offer minimal benefit for headache prevention. The antispasmodic drug tizanidine [Zanaflex] has shown some benefits in reducing chronic headaches in non-pregnant women; however, safety during pregnancy or nursing has not been evaluated and this drug should not be used when pregnant or breastfeeding.

Vitamins and Minerals

The American Academy of Pediatrics considers magnesium and riboflavin to be compatible with breastfeeding [8]; however, the safety of high-dose riboflavin used for migraine prevention has not been established. In general, preventive effects with these therapies are more modest than with prescription headache preventive treatments. Patients preferring to use nutritional supplements, however, may be offered magnesium while nursing.

> *Pearl for the practitioner:*
> Magnesium is compatible with breastfeeding, although efficacy as headache prevention is modest.

Summarizing Preventive Medication Recommendations

In general, non-medication preventive treatments should continue to be maximized during the period of lactation, especially therapies that have been shown to be consistently effective, such as stress management, relaxation, and biofeedback. Only some drugs within any drug category are listed among accepted safety recommendations, because of the low availability of literature to make safety determinations. Patients requiring medication therapy should limit treatment to propranolol, timolol, magnesium, and divalproex sodium (if consistent use of adequate contraception is ensured) (Table 7.2). Antidepressants should generally be avoided as headache preventive therapy, if possible.

Table 7.2 Preventive headache medications compatible with lactation

Medication	Dosage	Comments
Magnesium	600 mg QD	Watch for maternal diarrhea or stomach upset.
Divalproex sodium [Depakote]	Extended release: 500–1000 mg QD	Must ensure adequate contraception. Watch for maternal weight gain, bleeding, or hair thinning. Watch mom and infant for liver function and platelet count changes. Add daily folate.
Propranolol [Inderal]	Sustained release: 80–320 mg QD	Monitor baby for bradycardia, hypoglycemia, or cyanosis. Avoid in mothers prone to reactive airway disease.
Timolol [Blocadren]	10–15 mg BID	Monitor baby for bradycardia, hypoglycemia, or cyanosis. Avoid in mothers prone to reactive airway disease.
Verapamil [Calan]	Sustained release: 240 mg QD	Watch for maternal dizziness, constipation, or sedation. Monitor heart rate and blood pressure in the infant.

Atenolol should be limited, with monitoring for hypotension, bradycardia, tachypnea, and cyanosis in the baby. Avoid antidepressants, including amitriptyline [Elavil], bupropion [Wellbutrin], despiramine [Norpramin], doxepin [Sinequan], fluoxetine [Prozac], imipramine [Tofranil], nortriptyline [Pamelor], paroxetine [Paxil], sertraline [Zoloft], and trazadone [Desyrel].

Time Drug Administration to Minimize Effects

Using once-daily dosing can help minimize the baby's exposure by timing maternal dosing around the longest interval without nursing. In general, therefore, once-daily preventive therapies should be taken before the baby's longest period of sleep.

> *Pearl for the practitioner:*
> Once-daily preventive drugs should be administered before the baby's longest period of sleep.

Summary

During their final trimester of pregnancy patients should be prepared for the likely return of postpartum headaches with training in non-drug treatments and discussions about safe medication options after delivery. The beta-blockers propranolol and timolol offer the best efficacy and safety record when breast-feeding and should be considered first-line prevention therapies. Valproate may be used when breastfeeding only if reliable contraception is consistently used. The baby's exposure to maternal drugs may be reduced by timing the administration of daily prevention medication to precede the baby's longest sleep interval.

> *Practical pointers:*
> - Headaches recur postpartum in the majority of women.
> - Breastfeeding should be encouraged. Nursing is good for the newborn and likely will delay return of headaches in mom.
> - Non-drug approaches, such as stress management and relaxation techniques with or without biofeedback, are effective prevention therapies when breastfeeding.
> - More safe options for headache prevention are available for breast-feeding women than for pregnant women.
> - Recommended preventive drugs when nursing include propranolol, timolol, valproic acid (if adequate contraception can be ensured), and magnesium.

References

1. Taveras EM, Capra AM, Braveman PA, et al. Clinician support and psychosocial risk factors associated with breastfeeding discontinuation. *Pediatrics* 2003;112:108–115.
2. Sances G, Granella F, Nappi A, et al. Course of migraine during pregnancy and postpartum: a prospective study. *Cephalalgia* 2003;23:197–205.
3. Kennedy KI. Postpartum contraception. *Bailleres Clin Obste Gynaecol* 1996;10:25–41.
4. Sabers A. Pharmacokinetic interaction between contraceptives and antiepileptic drugs. *Seizure* 2008;17:141–144.
5. Topiramate (Topamax) for prevention of migraine. *Obstet Gynecol* 2005;105:1136–1137.

6. Marcus DA, Scharff L, Turk DC. Nonpharmacologial management of headaches during pregnancy. *Psychosom Med* 1995;57:527–535.
7. Scharff L, Marcus DA, Turk DC. Maintenance of effects in the nonmedical treatment of headaches during pregnancy. *Headache* 1996;36:285–290.
8. American Academy of Pediatric Committee on Drugs. The transfer of drugs and other chemicals into human milk. *Pediatrics* 2001;108:776–789.
9. Ostrea EM, Mantaring JB, Silvestre MA. Drugs that affect the fetus and newborn infant via the placenta or breast milk. *Pediatr Clin N Am* 2004;51:539–579.
10. Ohman I, Vitols S, Tomson T. Pharmacokinetics of gabapentin during delivery, in the neonatal period, and lactation: does a fetal accumulation occur during pregnancy? *Epilepsia* 2005;46:1621–1624.
11. Kristensen JH, Ilett KF, Hackett LP, Kohan R. Gabapentin and breastfeeding: a case report. *J Hum Lact* 2006;22:426–428.
12. Academy of Breastfeeding Medicine Protocol Committee. ABM clinical protocol #18: use of antidepressants in nursing mothers. *Breastfeed Med* 2008;3:44–52.

Chapter 8
Urgent Care/Emergency Treatment of the Acute, Severe Headache in Pregnant and Lactating Patients

Key Chapter Points

- Migraine is the #1 diagnosis of non-traumatic headache seen in the emergency department, accounting for 40–60% of all non-traumatic, emergency headaches.
- Emergency care of headache focuses on treatment of dehydration, nausea, and pain.
- Patients should rate their pain and nausea each using a visual analog scale from 0 (no symptoms) to 10 (severe symptoms). Target treatments that reduce both ratings to near zero to reduce the chance of headache recurrence.
- Non-drug treatments (e.g., ice packs, noise restriction, and light dimming) can substantially enhance symptomatic relief in the emergency room.
- The anti-emetic of choice for pregnant and lactating women is ondansetron.
- The pain medication treatments of choice for pregnant women include intravenous therapy with ketorolac (second trimester only), magnesium, or hydromorphone.
- The pain medication treatments of choice for lactating women include subcutaneous sumatriptan or intravenous therapy with ketorolac, valproate (provided that reliable contraception can be ensured), magnesium, or hydromorphone.
- Patients with residual headache after standard treatments may benefit from a greater occipital nerve block and/or a short course of prednisone.
- Since most emergency headaches are caused by recurring, primary headaches, follow-up care for future headache management is required.
- Written instructions enhance communication of post-discharge care and follow-up instructions.

Key words Acute migraine · Dehydration · Nausea · Non-traumatic

The lady in room three is a G2P1 in her 27th week of gestation. She was here five days ago for a severe headache, which was diagnosed as migraine. Even though we treated her with intravenous fluids, meperidine (Demerol), and metoclopramide (Reglan), she still said she had moderate severity pain when she left the ED. Now she's back with another

D.A. Marcus, P.A. Bain, *Effective Migraine Treatment in Pregnant and Lactating Women: A Practical Guide*, DOI 10.1007/978-1-60327-439-5_8, © Humana Press, a part of Springer Science+Business Media, LLC 2009

"headache." Since she's not getting any migraine treatment from a primary care doctor, I'm concerned that she may be a drug seeker.

Headache is one of the most common symptoms resulting in urgent care or emergency treatment. Using national statistics data about emergency service use, headache was the fourth most common reason for visiting an emergency department (ED), tied with back symptoms (Fig. 8.1) [1]. Headache accounted for 2.6% of all ED visits.

In most cases, non-traumatic head pain conditions seen in the ED are caused by primary, recurring headaches. In a prospective observational survey, discharge diagnoses were analyzed for all patients presenting to an ED with a chief complaint of non-traumatic headache over 11 months [2]. Migraine was the most common diagnosis (Table 8.1). Similarly, using data from the National Hospital Ambulatory Medical Care Survey, 2.1 million ED visits are made annually for non-traumatic headache, accounting for 2.2% of all ED visits [3]. In this survey,

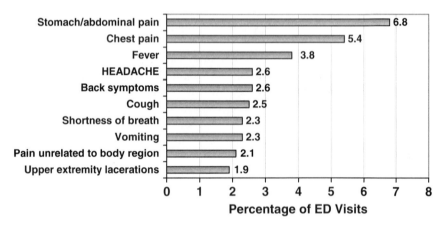

Fig. 8.1 Reasons for ED visits in the United States (Based on [1])

Table 8.1 Discharge diagnoses in consecutive ED patients with non-traumatic headache (Based on [2])

Diagnosis	Percentage
Migraine	41
Undifferentiated	37
Infection	10
Tension-type headache	4
Cluster headache	2
Stroke, transient ischemic attack, intracranial hemorrhage	2
Post-lumbar puncture headache	2
Benign intracranial hypertension (pseudotumor cerebri)	1
Glaucoma	1

migraine was again the most common single diagnosis, affecting two in every three patients treated in the ED for non-traumatic headache (63.5%). The next most common diagnoses were tension-type headache (3.4%), viral syndrome (2.4%), and anxiety/psychiatric diagnosis (1.1%). Twenty percent of headaches were diagnosed as "other benign conditions," including hypertension and infectious conditions affecting the ears, sinuses, throat, gastroenteritis or periapical abscess. Pathological diagnoses (including meningitis, encephalitis, stroke, hemorrhage, aneurysm, glaucoma, benign intracranial hypertension, giant cell/temporal arteritis, or hypertensive encephalopathy) were assigned to only 2% of headaches among all patients seen for non-traumatic headache. A pathological diagnosis was most common among older patients, accounting for 6% of non-traumatic headaches in patients $\geq$50 years old and 11% in those $\geq$75 years old. The evaluation for possible secondary headaches is detailed in Chapter 9.

> **Pearl for the practitioner:**
> While the vast majority of patients who present to the ER with non-traumatic headache will have migraine, other more ominous, though fortunately rare, causes of headache should be considered.

As seen in our case, headache treatment in the ED in both pregnant and non-pregnant patients generally relies on rehydration, analgesics, and anti-emetics. Review of 490 ED patients treated with parenteral medication for benign headache in three centers reported migraine as the most common diagnosis (58%), followed by non-specific headache (41%), and tension-type headache (1%) [4]. The most frequently used medications are shown in Table 8.2. Patients received an average of 2.1 different parenteral medications, with 82% of patients treated with at least two medications, 24% receiving at least three parenteral medications, and 7% treated with at least four parenteral drugs. Opioids were prescribed for almost half of all patients. A subanalysis of patients diagnosed with migraine similarly showed infrequent use of migraine-specific agents (dihydroergotamine in 6% and sumatriptan in 3%), with anti-emetics used for 49%, opioids for 44%, and ketorolac for 16%. A recent survey asking ED staff to identify first- and second-line ED treatment for migraine reported anti-emetics and parenteral non-steroidal anti-inflammatory drugs to be preferred first-line therapy, with opioids the preferred second-line treatment for patients failing first-line treatment [5]. Curiously, a minority of clinicians endorsed migraine-specific agents as first-line treatment (dihydroergotamine 9%; triptans 5%). The primary reasons for selecting anti-emetics or non-opioid analgesics as first-line therapy were treatment efficacy, drug availability in the ED, clinicians having received training in using these medications, and conformity with ED practice patterns.

While the studies described above refer to data for headache patients in general, many of the same doctrines can be applied to ED headaches in women during

Table 8.2 Most commonly used parenteral medications for benign headache in the ED (Based on [4])

Drug	Percentage of patients treated
Anti-emetic	
Prochloperazine	45.5
Diphenhydramine	36.6
Promethazine	22.7
Hydroxyzine	13.4
Droperidol	7.8
Metoclopramide	4.3
Analgesic	
Any opioid	47.6
Meperidine	35.6
Ketorolac	25.9
Migraine-specific drugs	
Sumatriptan	3.0
Dihydroergotamine	7.9
Glucocorticoids	
Dexamethasone	1.1
Methylprednisolone	0.5

pregnancy and lactation. In general, the emergency room/urgent care treatment of headaches is similar to drug therapy for non-emergency headaches. ED medication treatment during pregnancy and while nursing, however, will involve more limited choices to maximize safety for the baby. As in previous chapters, utilization of FDA pregnancy risk category classification and recommendations from the American Academy of Pediatrics [6] are used to help guide recommendations during pregnancy and lactation, respectively.

General principles for ED treatment of headache during pregnancy and lactation include:

- Utilize a consistent evaluation and treatment protocol for headache patients.
- Rule out secondary causes of headache.
- Treat dehydration.
- Treat nausea aggressively.
- Include non-medication treatments.
- Treat pain appropriately, reserving opioid medications for rescue therapy.
- Offer a short course of prednisone if headache pain is prolonged and fails to resolve (e.g., prednisone 20 mg twice daily for five days).
- Consider trigger point injections or occipital blocks.
- Arrange post-ED follow-up.

Applying each of these principles should help improve acute headache treatment and, as in the case of our patient still suffering in room three, minimize return visits for untreated or recurrent headache episodes.

Utilize a Consistent Evaluation and Treatment Plan

The ED evaluation of non-traumatic headache should utilize an organized approach to evaluation and treatment. As will be described in Chapter 9, secondary causes of headache should be ruled out by taking an appropriate history and performing a focused physical exam. Alarm symptoms should always be kept in mind. After secondary causes of headache are ruled out, a consistent sequence of treatment options is advised, including intravenous management with fluids, anti-nausea medications, and analgesics, as well as follow-up care instructions. Sample worksheets describing ED treatment of non-traumatic headache during pregnancy and lactation will be provided in this chapter to help facilitate efficient and consistent ED management. Employing protocols can further facilitate safe, efficient care for these patients in the ED and urgent care.

> *Pearl for the practitioner:*
> Develop and use a consistent evaluation and treatment strategy for pregnant and lactating patients who present to the ED for treatment of headaches. Pre-printed worksheets may help the clinician consider the full range of safe and effective available treatment options.

Rule Out Secondary Causes of Headache

As described in Chapter 1, headaches occurring during pregnancy may be caused by pathological conditions, most commonly:

- Pre-clampsia/Eclampsia;
- Stroke (both hemorrhagic and thrombotic);
- Arteriovenous malformations;
- Brain tumors (e.g., pituitary adenomas and meningiomas);
- Benign intracranial hypertension (formerly called pseudotumor cerebri);

While most patients seen in the ED with headache during pregnancy will have a primary or benign headache, examination should consider possible secondary headache conditions.

As with headaches occurring during pregnancy, postpartum headaches are also frequently caused by primary headaches. A review of 985 patients one week after delivery identified headache in 39% of women [7]. Two in every three headaches was diagnosed as tension-type or migraine headache (Fig. 8.2). Interestingly, only one in five women reporting a postural headache was diagnosed with a post-dural puncture headache; most postural headaches were also diagnosed as a primary headache disorder.

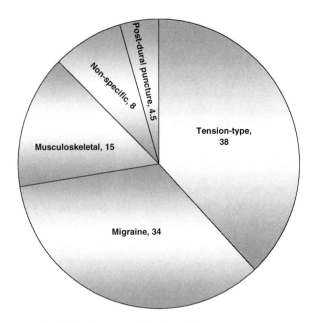

Fig. 8.2 Postpartum headache diagnoses (Based on [7])

Pearl for the practitioner:
Most non-traumatic headaches in the ER are due to migraine. Ominous secondary headaches, though rare, must be considered. The approach to the evaluation of possible secondary headaches is described in Chapter 9.

Treat Dehydration

Adequate hydration is particularly important for pregnant and lactating women. Maternal dehydration affects fetal amniotic fluid dynamics and may contribute to the development of oligohydramnios [8]. Although dehydration has been anecdotally linked to increased risk for pre-term labor, benefits from hydration for preventing pre-term labor are inconsistent [9]. Dehydration also increases the risk for thrombotic disorders, such as stroke, presumably because of increased viscosity [10].

Dehydration is linked to increased headache activity [11], while increasing water intake decreases headache severity and frequency [12]. Due to the frequent association of nausea and vomiting with headaches that result in an ED visit, the majority of ED headache patients will require rehydration.

> *Pearl for the practitioner:*
> Most patients who present to the ED for treatment of disabling headaches
> will be dehydrated. IV hydration is often very helpful.

Rehydration should occur with intravenous fluids. An interesting study using pregnant sheep detailed maternal and fetal effects of rehydration after dehydration using oral or intravenous maternal rehydration [13]. Arterial and urinary chemistry and hormonal levels, as well as cardiovascular markers, were assessed. Although maternal recovery occurred with either oral or intravenous rehydration, positive changes were seen early in the fetus only with maternal intravenous rehydration. While similar data evaluating rehydration in humans are not available, these data may support using intravenous dehydration as standard treatment for dehydration during pregnancy.

Treat Nausea Aggressively

In non-pregnant patients, anti-nausea medications help relieve both nausea and pain associated with severe migraine headaches in the ED. A retrospective chart review found that migraine pain was reduced by 3 or more points on a scale from 0 (no pain) to 10 (excruciating pain) 60% better with metoclopramide (Reglan) compared with hydromorphone (Dilaudid) (relative risk = 1.6) [14]. In another study, high dose metoclopramide (20 mg intravenously, redosed up to four times) was as effective as 6 mg of subcutaneous sumatriptan (Imitrex) [15]. Medications such as metoclopramide, prochlorperazine, and promethazine reduce headache pain and nausea because of their anti-dopaminergic activity. Akathisia, a feeling of inner restlessness, is a common side effect with dopaminergic anti-emetics.

These anti-nausea drugs have also demonstrated efficacy in reducing headache symptoms in non-pregnant patients, aside from their anti-emetic effects. In one study, 10 mg of prochloperazine (Compazine) was shown to be as effective as 20 mg of metoclopramide for the intravenous treatment of acute migraine, with both drugs administered in conjunction with 25 mg of intravenous diphenhydramine (Benadryl), an FDA risk category B drug [16]. Diphenhydramine, an antihistamine, has some antimigraine effects, promotes helpful sedation, and counteracts akathisia that often accompanies drugs affecting dopamine. In other studies, intramuscular droperidol (Inapsine) was more effective in relieving headache-related pain than prochloperazine [17] and as effective as meperidine (Demerol) [18]. Unfortunately, while droperidol is an excellent medication for nausea and headache pain, it has been associated with cases of QT prolongation. The FDA has issued a black box warning emphasizing this risk. Because of this, use of droperidol should be restricted, if it is used at all.

Recently, the combination of trimethobenzamide (Tigan, FDA risk category C) plus diphenhydramine (Benadryl, FDA risk category B) was compared with sumatriptan (FDA risk category C) for ED treatment of acute migraine in non-pregnant patients [19]. While short-term relief was superior with sumatriptan, anti-nausea therapy offered similar 24-hour relief, and the authors suggested that anti-nausea therapy may provide an appropriate acute ED therapy for patients unable to use sumatriptan. As trimethobenzamide and sumatriptan are FDA risk category C medications, other, safer alternatives should be considered first for nausea and pain.

Anti-emetics most commonly prescribed by practicing obstetricians are promethazine (Phenergan) and ondansetron (Zofran) [20] (See Table 8.3). Metoclopramide (Reglan) and prochlorperazine (Compazine) may also be used. Many women treated with intravenous metoclopramide or prochlorperazine develop akathisia, which may not be appreciated unless specifically asked about. If present, this requires additional treatment with intravenous diphenhydramine (Benadryl). Although trimethobenzamide (Tigan) is an FDA pregnancy risk category C drug, limited human data have suggested possible increased risk of

Table 8.3 ED medications for headache during pregnancy

Drug	FDA Class	Dose	Comments
Anti-emetics			
Ondansetron (Emeset, Emetron, Ondemet, Zofran)	B	4–8 mg IV over 2–5 minutes. May use IM if poor venous access.	Well tolerated. Preferred by obstetricians.
Metoclopramide* (Reglan)	B	10–20 mg IV	More effective than hydromorphone alone [41]. Metoclopramide 20 mg IV shown to be as effective as SQ sumatriptan (Imitrex) [15]. Watch for akathisia.
Promethazine (Phenergan, Promethegan)	C	12.5–25 mg IM	Both anti-emetic and antihistamine components may improve migraine. Watch for akathisia.
Droperidol (Inapsine)	C	2.5–5 mg IM	May be more effective in relieving headache pain than prochlorperazine [17]. As effective as opioid [18]. Black box warning for QT prolongation; not recommended.
Prochlorperazine* (Compazine)	C	10 mg IV	As effective as metoclopramide (Reglan) [16]. Watch for akathisia.
Trimethobenzamide* (Tigan)	C	200 mg IM	Limited human data suggest possible increased risk of congenital anomalies. Use cautiously.

Table 8.3 (continued)

Drug	FDA Class	Dose	Comments
Pain medications			
Magnesium sulfate	B	1–2 g IV	As effective as metoclopramide [27].
Tramadol (Ultram)	C	100 mg IM	Similar efficacy to IM NSAID in non-pregnant patients [23]. Not readily available at all centers.
Hydromorphone (Dilaudid)	C	1–2 mg IM or SQ 0.5–1 mg IV over 2–3 minutes	Avoid prolonged use. Use at term may result in neonatal respiratory depression.
Dexamethasone	C	4–10 mg IV	Minimal efficacy in typical acute migraine; beneficial for migraine lasting >72 hours [34].

*FDA risk category B drug diphenhydramine (Benadryl) may be administered as 25 mg IV in patients experiencing restlessness after receiving anti-emetics.
IM=intramuscular; IV=intravenous; SQ=subcutaneous.

congenital anomalies with trimethobenzamide exposure, supporting cautious and limited use during pregnancy. Ondansetron is, consequently, preferred for nausea treatment, due to the superior tolerability (e.g., less akathisia and sedation) and its designation as an FDA risk category B drug. As described in Chapter 5, ondansetron is also preferred during breastfeeding [21]. Availability as a generic product has reduced cost constraints with ondansetron.

> **Pearl for the practitioner:**
> Ondansetron is the preferred ED anti-emetic during pregnancy or lactation and can be administered intravenously or intramuscularly when venous access is limited.

Always Consider Non-medication Treatments

As described in Chapter 3, non-medication therapies provide effective and safe treatment options as monotherapy or adjunctive treatment. Unfortunately, these common sense measures are often overlooked in the busy ED. Routinely incorporating non-drug treatments can improve patient comfort and treatment satisfaction [22].

Headache-provoking external stimulation can be decreased by reducing lighting and limiting noise, as well as offering soothing music and ice packs. Placing the headache patient immediately in a darkened, quiet exam room, away from the commotion of the busy ED and quickly offering an ice pack are easy ways to help the patient and show compassion. Trained ED staff who perform relaxation exercises, neck massage, and gentle cervical range of motion exercises can substantially enhance the efficacy of other headache-relieving therapies administered during the ED visit.

> **Pearl for the practitioner:**
> While simple common sense measures such as putting the headache patient in a darkened, quiet room and offering an ice pack are useful and appreciated by patients, they are often overlooked in a busy ED.

Treat Pain Appropriately

Studies are not available that have directly assessed ED treatment in pregnant women. Indeed, pregnancy is generally an exclusion in clinical trials assessing ED therapies. Analgesics are effective for treating migraine in the ED in non-pregnant patients [23], and may be used when appropriate during pregnancy and breastfeeding (Table 8.3). Often useful non-opioid treatment options are overlooked and ED clinicians move quickly to opioids, which can result in undesirable effects, including side effects and inadvertently promoting repeat ED visits or drug-seeking behavior.

Nonsteroidal anti-inflammatory drugs are typically limited to the second trimester of pregnancy [24]. Intravenous ketorolac can be safely used while nursing because of a low milk-to-plasma ratio [6]. In a prospective, double-blind study, 30 mg of intravenous ketorolac (Toradol) was shown to be more effective than intranasal sumatriptan [25]. In one study, a 100 mg infusion of tramadol (Ultram) in 100 mL saline, administered over 30 minutes, effectively treated migraine in the ED. Tramadol is an FDA risk category C drug. The effects of tramadol in the nursing baby are unknown, although both the parent drug and its active metabolite are excreted into breast milk. Consequently, women needing to use tramadol while lactating should pump and discard milk after exposure, supplementing the next feeding with stored milk.

> **Pearl for the practitioner:**
> Limit nonsteroidal anti-inflammatory drugs, like intravenous ketorolac, to the second trimester of pregnancy. Ketorolac is compatible with nursing and is a good first-line treatment because of its low milk-to-plasma ratio.

Intravenous magnesium sulfate may also be used in the ED treatment of migraine, with efficacy shown using 1 g intravenously [26]. It is an FDA risk category B drug, safe in both pregnancy and lactation. In a randomized prospective study, 2 g of intravenous magnesium sulfate was as effective as 10 mg of intravenous metoclopramide and more effective than placebo [27].

> ***Pearl for the practitioner:***
> 1–2 mg intravenous magnesium sulfate may safely and effectively treat
> ED migraine in pregnant and lactating women.

Nursing patients can also be treated with subcutaneous sumatriptan, which has a long track record of reliable efficacy as an emergency treatment for severe headache. In a pilot study comparing headache relief with 3 mg versus 6 mg of subcutaneous sumatriptan, treatment efficacy was similar with both doses although patients preferred the 3 mg dose [28]. Intravenous sodium valproate (Depacon) can alternatively be used in patients with reliable contraception [29]. Dilute intravenous valproate is typically administered by an infusion over 5–15 minutes, although efficacy benefits have been inconsistent [30]. A small study treating 40 non-pregnant patients with typical migraine intravenously with 500 mg of valproate versus 10 mg of prochlorperazine, each diluted in 10 mL of saline and administered over 2 minutes, showed better success with prochlorperazine, with additional rescue therapy required in 79% treated with valproate versus 25% with prochlorperazine [31].

> ***Pearl for the practitioner:***
> Though not recommended during pregnancy, subcutaneous sumatriptan
> may be safely used when lactating.

Despite the fact that opioids offer only modest benefit for migraine relief, a survey of 500 randomly-selected ED charts from patients with a primary diagnosis of migraine showed opioids to be the most commonly prescribed first-line ED treatment (60% of patients) [32]. This over-reliance on opioids as ED treatment is particularly problematic in non-pregnant patients, for whom triptans offer clearly superior efficacy. Although intramuscular opioids are easy to administer in an ED, treating headache or other chronic pain with this class of medications can lead to frequent return visits for more opioids. Opioids may have a greater role in pregnant patients whose access to effective migraine-specific treatments like triptans and dihydroergotamine is restricted. Opioids may be used as rescue therapy, although a recent study showed that migraine patients treated with opioids in the ED had longer duration visits compared with patients treated with non-opioids, further supporting cautious use in patients with benign headache [33]. Although frequently used to treat migraine in the ED, meperidine (Demerol) should be avoided because of potential risks with accumulation of metabolites, such as normeperidine. For this reason, alternative opioids, such as hydromorphone (Dilaudid), are preferred.

> *Pearl for the practitioner:*
> If parenteral opioids are needed as rescue therapy, avoid meperidine and use hydromorphone instead.

Dexamethasone (Decadron) has minimal efficacy in most patients receiving ED treatment of migraine, although benefit has been shown in patients with migraine lasting >72 hours [34]. In a recent study, dexamethasone treatment in ED migraine patients was shown to be ineffective for preventing migraine relapse [35]. Furthermore, dexamethasone crosses the placenta and is not preferred in pregnancy. Prednisone is an FDA risk category B drug, and may be used as rescue therapy when acute ED treatment has failed and disabling migraine is prolonged and unremitting [36]. Providing a short course of prednisone (e.g., 20 mg twice daily for 5 days) can help resolve a prolonged, non-responsive headache episode.

Intranasal lidocaine (FDA risk category B) administered as a 4% solution with the patient lying down with the head hyper-extended may be used to effectively treat patients with recalcitrant cluster headaches. Randomized, controlled trials using intranasal lidocaine for acute or ED treatment of migraine, however, have produced inconsistent results [37,38]. Anecdotally, intranasal lidocaine has been effective and can be a safer useful option for headache treatment.

Consider Trigger Point Injections or Occipital Blocks

Chapter 6 describes the benefits of trigger point injections or occipital nerve blocks for temporary relief and prevention of recalcitrant headaches in pregnant women. These blocks have been used to successfully treat primary headaches in the ED [39]. Blocks can provide a safe and effective way to break a prolonged headache cycle. This procedure can easily be learned by ER and urgent care personnel. For women who are far along in their pregnancy, it is often more comfortable for them to be leaning over with their head on the exam table during the procedure, rather than to be in the prone position.

> *Pearl for the practitioner:*
> Occipital nerve blocks are another safe, effective treatment option that can be performed in the ED and/or urgent care clinic.

Doctors from Kaiser Permanente in Santa Rosa, CA presented data at the American Headache Society scientific meeting in 2005, describing benefits from three possible non-sedating rescue therapies in patients who had failed initial headache therapy [40]. A total of 197 patients with benign headache (including nine pregnant women) were treated with rescue therapy with either oxygen by face mask at 10 L/minute, a dental discluder (BestBite™), or bilateral greater occipital nerve blocks using 2 mL of 0.5% bupivicaine. Average pain reductions were 43% with oxygen, 46% with the dental device, and 56% with occipital nerve blocks. Substantial pain reduction was achieved most consistently with occipital nerve blocks, regardless of headache diagnosis.

Arrange Post-ED Follow-up

Migraines recur within 48 hours in one in ten to one in three patients successfully treated for acute migraine in the ED [23,41]. Therefore, arranging post-ED follow-up is essential to maximize the development of a safe and effective long-term headache management plan. As seen by our patient in room three, failure to provide a clear post-discharge plan for persistent or recurrent headache may result in repeat ED visits. Patients are often groggy after headache treatment (which may also be part of the postdrome phase of the headache) and may not be able to accurately understand or remember follow-up recommendations. Communicating post-ED treatment recommendations can be enhanced by providing clear, easy-to-understand written after-care instructions. Primary headaches are most effectively managed with good outpatient support and follow-up, providing patients with both non-medication options and medications they can administer at home, rather than waiting for headache severity and disability to increase and precipitate a repeat ED visit. Providing a written treatment strategy that can be modified at the follow-up visit in their headache provider's office can empower the patients by giving them an organized approach to treating acute episodes.

Unfortunately, despite the recurrent nature of most non-traumatic headaches seen in the ED, most patients, like our case, receive limited recommendations for the treatment of recurring or future headaches or follow-up care plans. A survey of patients receiving ED treatment for a chief complaint of headache reported that only 22% were pain-free on discharge, with mild pain in 42% and moderate to severe pain in the remainder [42]. Discharge medications were provided to only 37% of patients. Migraine was the most common diagnosis, which would typically be expected to recur. Headache returned within 24 hours in two of three patients. Unfortunately, only 41% of patients were advised to arrange follow-up with a physician for headache management. Lack of follow-up planning supports the need to more effectively eliminate nausea and head pain symptoms during the ED visit with effective therapies. Furthermore, consistently arranging follow-up care offers a significant opportunity to reduce the need for future ED headache care.

> *Pearl for the practitioner:*
> Expect headaches to recur in most patients presenting to the ED with primary headache. Patients will therefore need clear (and, ideally) written post-discharge treatment recommendations and plans for follow-up.

Boxes 8.1–8.3 provide simple post-ED instruction sheets, along with suggestions for appropriate ED and post-discharge instructions for women during pregnancy and lactation. A summary of preferred ED headache treatments during pregnancy and lactation is provided in Table 8.4.

Box 8.1 ED discharge instructions for headache patient

You were just treated for an acute headache episode. You will need to follow up with your primary care provider for ongoing care of your headaches. Please make an appointment to be seen within the next 2 weeks.

You were prescribed a small amount of medication to treat your symptoms if they return:

For nausea
___metoclopramide
___prochlorperazine
___ondansetron
___other_____

For pain
___acetaminophen
___other_____

Contact your primary care provider if additional medication is needed.

Box 8.2 ED headache treatment options during pregnancy

- Urgent care/ED treatments
  - Ice pack, massage, neck stretches
  - Reduced lights, reduced noise, soothing music
  - Intravenous rehydration
  - Anti-emetic

    □ IV ondansetron (Zofran) 4–8 mg over 2–5 minutes
    □ IM promethazine (Phenergan) 12.5–25 mg, with monitoring for akathisia
    □ IV/IM prochlorperazine (Compazine) 5–10 mg (over 5 minutes if IV), with monitoring for akathisia

  - Analgesic

    □ Hydromorphone (Dilaudid) 1–2 mg IM/SQ or 0.5-1 mg IV over 2–3 minutes
    □ Occipital nerve blocks
    □ Trigger point injections

- Discharge medication recommendations
  - Anti-emetic

    - □ Zofran 4–8 mg ½–1 tablet every 6 hours as needed for severe nausea (Patients may prefer orally dissolvable tablet)
    - □ Compazine 10 mg PO every 6 hours as needed
    - □ Compazine 25 mg PR every 6 hours as needed
  - Analgesic

    - □ Acetaminophen 650 mg PO/PR every 6 hours as needed
    - □ Hydrocodone 10 mg (Vicodin, Norco) PO ½–1 tablet every 6 hours as needed (Prescribe no more than 15 tablets.)
  - Rescue therapy

    - □ Prednisone 20 mg tablet PO twice daily for 5 days

IM = intramuscular; IV = intravenous; PO = oral; PR = rectal; SQ = subcutaneous

Box 8.3 ED headache treatment options during lactation

- Urgent care/ED treatments
  - Ice pack, massage, neck stretches
  - Reduced lights, reduced noise, soothing music
  - Intravenous rehydration
  - Anti-emetic

    - □ IV ondansetron (Zofran) 4–8 mg over 2–5 minutes
  - Analgesic

    - □ Ketorolac (Toradol) 30 mg IV or 60 mg IM
    - □ SQ sumatriptan (Imitrex) 3–6 mg (Efficacy is similar with 3 and 6 mg, with patients preferring the lower dosage.)
    - □ IV sodium valproate (Depacon) 500 mg diluted in 10 mL saline and administered over 5–15 minutes if reliable contraception is ensured
    - □ Hydromorphone (Dilaudid) 1–2 mg IM/SQ or 0.5–1.0 mg IV over 2–3 minutes every 2 hours, as needed
    - □ Occipital nerve blocks
    - □ Trigger point injections
    - □ IV dexamethasone (Decadron) 4 mg

- Discharge medication recommendations
  - Anti-emetic

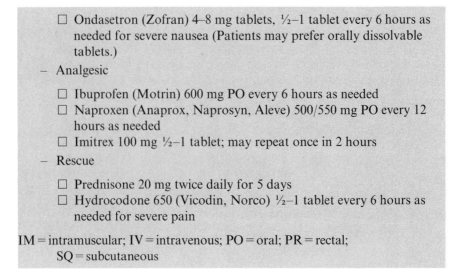

      ☐ Ondasetron (Zofran) 4–8 mg tablets, ½–1 tablet every 6 hours as needed for severe nausea (Patients may prefer orally dissolvable tablets.)
- Analgesic

      ☐ Ibuprofen (Motrin) 600 mg PO every 6 hours as needed
      ☐ Naproxen (Anaprox, Naprosyn, Aleve) 500/550 mg PO every 12 hours as needed
      ☐ Imitrex 100 mg ½–1 tablet; may repeat once in 2 hours
- Rescue

      ☐ Prednisone 20 mg twice daily for 5 days
      ☐ Hydrocodone 650 (Vicodin, Norco) ½–1 tablet every 6 hours as needed for severe pain

IM = intramuscular; IV = intravenous; PO = oral; PR = rectal; SQ = subcutaneous

Table 8.4 Preferred treatment of headache in the ED

	Pregnancy	Lactation
First-line	Non-medication therapies	Non-medication therapies
	Rehydration	Rehydration
	Ondansetron (Zofran)	Ketorolac (Toradol)
	Ketorolac (Toradol)—2nd trimester only	Sumatriptan (Imitrex)
		Odansetron (Zofran)
Second-line	Magnesium sulfate	Magnesium sulfate
	Tramadol (Ultram)	
Other	Hydromorphone (Dilaudid)	Valproate (Depacon)
	Intranasal lidocaine	Hydromorphone (Dilaudid)
	Occipital nerve blocks	Occipital nerve blocks
	Trigger point injections	Trigger point injections

Summary

The majority of patients seen in the ER for non-traumatic headache will be diagnosed with migraine, with secondary headaches more common in older adults. ED headache treatment during pregnancy and lactation focuses on intravenous rehydration and nausea management with ondansetron. Residual pain treatments differ in women who are pregnant or nursing, although safer options are available. Due to the recurrent nature of most headaches seen in the ED, treatment should include clear, written discharge instructions, including recommendations for outpatient headache management care.

Practical pointers

- While migraine is the most common etiology of headaches seen in the ED, ominous, though fortunately more rare, secondary causes of headache should be considered.
- Most ED headache patients will be dehydrated and require intravenous hydration.
- Treatment efficacy can be enhanced by employing simple, non-drug headache-relieving strategies, including promptly admitting the patient to a dark, quiet room and offering an ice pack.
- Nausea should be treated aggressively, with ondansetron preferred during pregnancy and lactation. Ondasetron can be administered intravenously, or intramuscularly if venous access is difficult to obtain.
- Appropriate pain management includes ketorolac during the second trimester of pregnancy and when lactating. Intravenous magnesium can be used during pregnancy or when nursing. Sumatriptan may also be used in lactating women. Opioids should be reserved as rescue therapy when other treatments are ineffective.
- If opioids are necessary, hydromorphone is preferred.
- Additional rescue therapies may include occipital nerve blocks or a short course of prednisone.
- Discharge instructions should include recommendations for treating recurring nausea and headache, as well as outpatient follow-up care.

References

1. McCaig LF, Nawar EW. National Hospital Ambulatory Medical Care Survey. 2004 emergency department summary. *Adv Data* 2006;372:1–29.
2. Fiesseler FW, Riggs RL, Holubek W, Eskin B, Richman PB. Canadian Headache Society criteria for the diagnosis of acute migraine headache in the ED – do our patients meet these criteria? *Am J Emerg Med* 2005;23:149–154.
3. Goldstein JN, Camargo CA, Pelletier AJ, Edlow JA. Headache in the United States emergency departments: demographics, work-up and frequency of pathological disease. *Cephalalgia* 2006;26:684–690.
4. Vinson DR, Hurtado TR, Vandenberg JT, Banwart L. Variations among emergency departments in the treatment of benign headache. *Ann Emerg Med* 2003;41:90–97.
5. Hurtado TR, Vinson DR, Vandenberg JT. ED treatment of migraine headache: factors influencing pharmacotherapeutic choices. *Headache* 2007;47:1134–1143.
6. American Academy of Pediatric Committee on Drugs. The transfer of drugs and other chemicals into human milk. *Pediatrics* 2001;108:776–789.
7. Goldszmidt E, Chettle C, Kern R, et al. The incidence and etiology of postpartum headaches. *Can J Anesth* 2004;51:A59.
8. Schreyer P, Sherman DJ, Ervin MG, Day L, Ross MG. Maternal dehydration: impact on ovine amniotic fluid volume and composition. *J Dev Physiol* 1990;13:283–287.
9. Urbanski PK. How does hydration affect preterm labor? *AWHONN Lifelines* 1997;1:25.

10. Skidmore FM, Williams LS, Fradkin KD, Alonso RJ, Biller J. Presentation, etiology, and outcome of stroke in pregnancy and puerperium. *J Stroke Cerebrovasc Dis* 2001;10: 1–10.
11. Blau JN. Water deprivation: a new migraine precipitant. *Headache* 2005;45:757–759.
12. Spigt MG, Kuijper EC, Schayck CP, et al. Increasing daily water intake for prophylactic treatment of headache: a pilot trial. *Eur J Neurol* 2005;12:715–718.
13. Agnew CL, Ross MG, Fujino Y, et al. Maternal/fetal dehydration: prolonged effects and responses to oral hydration. *Am J Physiol* 1993;264:R197–R203.
14. Griffith JD, Mycyck MB, Kyriacou DN. Metoclopramide versus hydrocodone for the emergency department treatment of migraine headache. *J Pain* 2008;88–94.
15. Friedman BW, Corbo J, Lipton RB. A trial of metoclopramide vs sumatriptan for the emergency department treatment of migraines. *Neurology* 2005;64:463–468.
16. Friedman BW, Esses D, Solorzano C, et al. A randomized controlled trial of prochloperazine versus metoclopramide for treatment of acute migraine. *Ann Emerg Med* 2008;52:399–406.
17. Miner JR, Fish SJ, Smith SW, Biros MH. Droperidol vs. prochloperazine for benign headaches in the emergency department. *Acad Emerg Med* 2001;8:873–879.
18. Richman PB, Allegra J, Eskin B, et al. A randomized clinical trial to assess the efficacy of intramuscular droperidol for the treatment of acute migraine. *Am J Emerg Med* 2002;20:39–42.
19. Friedman BW, Hockberg M, Esses D, et al. A clinical trial of trimethobenzamide/ diphenhydramine versus sumatriptan for acute migraine. *Headache* 2006;46:934–941.
20. Power ML, Milligan LA, Schulkin J. Managing nausea and vomiting of pregnancy: a survey of obstetrician-gynecologists. *J Reprod Med* 2007;52:922–928.
21. Mahadevan U, Kane S. American Gastroenterological Association Institute Medical Position Statement on the Use of Gastrointestinal Medications in Pregnancy. *Gastroenterology* 2006;131:283–311.
22. Dillard JN, Knapp S. Complementary and alternative pain therapy in the emergency department. *Emerg Med Clin North Am* 2005;23:529–549.
23. Engindeniz Z, Demircan C, Karli N, et al. Intramuscular tramadol vs. Diclofenac sodium for the treatment of acute migraine attacks in emergency departments: a prospective, randomised, double-blind study. *J Headache Pain* 2005;6:143–148.
24. Evers S, Áfra J, Frese A, et al. EFNS guideline on the drug treatment of migraine – report of an EFNS task force. *Eur J Neurol* 2006;13:560–572.
25. Meredith JT, Wait S, Brewer KL. A prospective double-blind study of nasal sumatriptan versus IV ketorolac in migraine. *Am J Emerg Med* 2003;21:173–175.
26. Bigal ME, Bordini CA, Tepper SJ, Speciali JG. Intrvenous magnesium sulphate in the acute treatment of migraine without aura and migraine with aura. A randomized, double-blind, placebo-controlled study. *Cephalalgia* 2002;22:345–353.
27. Cete Y, Dora B, Ertan C, Ozdemir C, Oktay C. A randomized prospective placebo-controlled study of intravenous magnesium sulphate vs. metoclopramide in the management of acute migraine attacks in the Emergency Department. *Cephalalgia* 2005;25:199–204.
28. Landy SH, McGinnis JE, McDonald SA. Pilot study evaluating preference for 3-mg versus 6-mg subcutaneous sumatriptan. *Headache* 2005;45:346–349.
29. Waberzinek G, Marková, Mastík J. Safety and efficacy of intravenous sodium valproate in the treatment of acute migraine. *Neuro Endocrinol Lett* 2007;28:59–64.
30. Frazee LA, Foraker KC. Use of intravenous valproic acid for acute migraine. *Ann Pharmacother* 2008;42:403–407.
31. Tanen DA, Miller S, French T, Riffenburgh RH. Intravenous sodium valproate versus prochloperazine for the emergency department treatment of acute migraine headaches: a prospective, randomized, double-blind trial. *Ann Emerg Med* 2003;41:847–853.
32. Colman I, Rothney A, Wright SC, Zilkalns B, Rowe BH. Use of narcotic analgesics in the emergency department treatment of migraine headache. *Neurology* 2004;62: 1695–1700.

33. Tornabene SV, Deutsch R, Davis DP, Chan TC, Vilke GM. Evaluating the use and timing of opioids for the treatment of migraine headaches in the emergency department. *J Emerg Med*, in press.

34. Friedman BW, Greenwald P, Bania TC, et al. Randomized trial of IV dexamethasone for acute migraine in the emergency department. *Neurology* 2007;69:2038–2044.

35. Rowe BH, Colman I, Edmonds ML, et al. Randomized controlled trial of intravenous dexamethasone to prevent relapse in acute migraine headache. *Headache* 2008;48: 333–340.

36. Von Seggern RL, Adelman JU: Practice and economics cost considerations in headache treatment. Part 2: acute migraine treatment. *Headache* 1996;36:493–502.

37. Maizels M, Geiger AM. Intranasal lidocaine for migraine: a randomized trial and open-label follow-up. *Headache* 1999;39:543–551.

38. Blanda M, Rench T, Gerson LW, Weigand JV. Intranasal lidocaine for the treatment of migraine headache: a randomized, controlled trial. *Acad Emerg Med* 2001;8:337–342.

39. Scattoni L, Di Stani F, Villani V, et al. Great occipital nerve blockade for cluster headache in the emergency department: case report. *J Headache Pain* 2006;7:98–100.

40. Bernstein AL, Morgan BG, Ho JK. A drop-in headache clinic for acute headaches. The value of early intervention with non-sedating modalities. *Headache* 2005;45:832 [abstract].

41. Innes GD, Macphail I, Dillon EC, Metcalfe C, Gao M. Dexamethasone prevents relapse after emergency department treatment of acute migraine: a randomized clinical trial. *CJEM* 1999;1:26–33.

42. Gupta MX, Silberstein SD, Young WB, et al. Less is not more: underutilization of headache medications in a university hospital emergency department. *Headache* 2007;47:1125–1133.

Chapter 9
Work-up for Headache During Pregnancy and Lactation

Key Chapter Points

- Most headaches seen in the emergency department are primary headaches. Secondary headaches, though less common, need to be considered.
- Patients with new onset headache or a change in headache pattern should be evaluated for possible secondary headaches.
- Patient history and physical examination will usually provide adequate information to determine headache diagnosis.
- A spinal fluid examination is safe and reliable during pregnancy, with normal values comparable to those in non-pregnant adults.
- Neuroimaging should be performed during pregnancy if medically indicated and if the results may change treatment during pregnancy.
- Neuroimaging contrast agents can be safely used if necessary during pregnancy and lactation.

Keywords Lumbar puncture · Magnetic resonance imaging · Spinal fluid

This 24-year-old G1P0 in her 12th gestational week with an otherwise uncomplicated pregnancy presented to a local emergency department for evaluation and treatment of severe headaches. She had a history of migraine headaches and her physical exam was normal. Because of this, her headaches were thought to be migraine. She was referred from the emergency department to the neurology service for participation in a research study evaluating the benefits of biofeedback in chronic headaches during pregnancy. She was seen by the neurologist the following day and noted to be ill-appearing and covering her eyes. She reported marked photophobia and pain with moving her eyes. She was flushed and her skin was hot to the touch. She was febrile with a temperature of 102 degrees Fahrenheit, a heart rate of 110, and normal blood pressure. Though she reported a prior history of migraine headaches, her current headaches were quite different. She was sent back to the emergency department where a spinal tap was performed and the diagnosis of viral meningitis was confirmed.

In this patient's case, the previous diagnosis of migraine, normal neurological examination, and desire by the emergency staff to provide safe, non-medication treatment during pregnancy may have resulted in a delayed diagnosis of a

D.A. Marcus, P.A. Bain, *Effective Migraine Treatment in Pregnant and Lactating Women: A Practical Guide*, DOI 10.1007/978-1-60327-439-5_9, © Humana Press, a part of Springer Science+Business Media, LLC 2009

secondary headache. As in non-pregnant patients, new headaches or a significant change in headache activity during pregnancy requires an evaluation to differentiate benign primary headaches from pathological headaches. Headache associated with papilledema, focal neurological signs or symptoms, loss of consciousness, or seizures suggests intracranial pathology and requires a thorough history and complete medical and neurological evaluations. Fortunately, most cases of new onset headaches during pregnancy are primary headaches, such as migraine and tension-type. Less common but more ominous secondary headaches, however, should always be considered.

> **Pearl for the practitioner:**
> The vast majority of headaches in pregnant women are primary migraine or tension-type headaches. Rare, more ominous secondary headaches must be considered.

Transient neurological symptoms, such as migraine aura, may also develop during pregnancy. During a two-year period, 41 patients who developed transient neurological symptoms during pregnancy were evaluated [1]. Migraine with aura was the predominant diagnosis ($N = 34$, 83%). Additional diagnoses in two patients were stroke and carpal tunnel syndrome, and in one patient presyncope from anemia, multiple sclerosis, and epilepsy were noted. Patients were followed yearly for five years with no reports of cerebrovascular episodes in any patient during that time. Although this study showed that transient neurological symptoms occurring during pregnancy were typically migraine-related, all women developing a new or worsening of a typical migraine aura or other transient neurological symptoms should have a thorough history and detailed medical and neurological evaluations.

The work-up of suspected secondary headaches includes a thorough history, a focused physical and neurological exam, and, at times, specialized testing such as spinal fluid examination and/or brain imaging. This chapter will provide an overview of the secondary headache evaluation, and provide recommendations regarding indications for specialized testing during pregnancy and lactation.

Headache History

Patients presenting with a complaint of new headache or change in headache pattern should be questioned about their general health, as well as headache activity. A series of questions can be used to help determine both a likely preliminary diagnosis and the need for additional testing (Box 9.1). Always ask patients to identify how many different types of headaches they have. If they have more than one headache, ask them to answer questions for their most severe and their mildest headache separately. Often patients

Box 9.1 Questions to be answered by new headache patients (Adapted from Marcus DA. Chronic pain. A primary care guide to practical management. 2nd edition, Humana Press, Totowa, NJ, 2008.)

1. How long have your headaches been the way they are now?
   If new or change in headache occurred within past 2 years, consider more extensive evaluation.

2. Do you have one type of headache or more?
   If >1 type, ask questions to identify each type of headache.

3. Does your headache occur intermittently, or do you always have head pain?
   Ask about frequent prescription or over-the-counter analgesic use if daily.

4. How often do you get your headache?
   Frequent headaches may be due to analgesic overuse or may signal a secondary headache.

5. How long does each headache episode typically last?
   Headaches lasting <2 hours may indicate cluster headache, though this is an uncommon diagnosis in women of childbearing age. Migraines usually last 4–72 hours. Also, the time course of headache may dictate therapy: short-acting medications are best for headaches that reach maximum intensity quickly; long-acting medications are often needed for headaches lasting ≥12 hours.

6. What do you typically do when you have a headache?
   a. Are usual activities reduced or curtailed?
   b. Do you go to bed?
   c. Do you need to turn off the television, radio, or lights in the room?
   Headache-related disability or sensitivity to noise or lights suggest migraine.

7. Are you having a headache right now? If so, is this how severe your headaches usually get, or is this an especially "good" or "bad" day?
   Patient behavior in the clinic can be compared with historical reports if the patient is having a typical headache during the examination.

8. Where is the pain located? Is it always in the same location?
   Headache pain typically shifts among various areas on the head during different headache episodes. Pain that is always located in the same spot (with the exception of cluster headache, which usually involves the same eye with each episode) or is located in the back of the head or neck often requires additional work-up.

9. Any other new problems since the headache began?

Identification of new medical (e.g., fever, weight loss, or other constitutional or system complaints) or neurological symptoms will suggest the need for additional evaluations.

10. Do you have family members with similar headaches?
    Migraine headaches often run in families. If one parent has migraine, his or her child has a 50% chance of developing migraines. If both parents have migraine headaches, this risk increases to 75%.

who report >2 different headaches actually have only one or two unique types of headache, with differences in severity interpreted by the patient as separate headache disorders.

Red Flags/Alarm Symptoms

Alteration in headache pattern unrelated to change in medication, exposures, etc., is often cause for a more detailed evaluation. Any new headache, whether mild or severe, is important to assess. Although patients often worry that their headaches may be caused by brain tumors, most patients presenting with headache related to brain tumor have a variety of neurological complaints, including mental status or cognitive changes as well as focal neurological deficits. Headache is usually not the most prominent presenting symptom in patients ultimately diagnosed with brain tumors.

Taking a thorough headache-related history can help to identify red flags that may signify a secondary headache, including common causes of pathologic headache, like infection and trauma (Box 9.2). Several clinical characteristics have been associated with serious intracranial pathology [2]:

- New onset headache or significant change in headache character within two years;
- Posterior head or neck pain;
- Patient ≥50 years of age;
- Abnormal neurological examination.

Patients with red flags or any of the four features suggesting possible intracranial pathology will require more detailed evaluation. Additional alarm symptoms that warrant more detailed examination include seizures, loss of consciousness, fever, and weight loss.

Pearl for the practitioner:
Clinicians need to evaluate patients for possible red flag signs and symptoms that may suggest significant underlying pathology and secondary headaches.

Box 9.2 Red flags suggesting need for additional work-up

- Trauma
- Fever
- Seizures
- Loss of consciousness
- Change in previously stable headache pattern
- History of malignancy
- Neurological symptoms or signs
- Unexplained weight loss
- Age >50 years

Physical Examination

Focused, but thorough, general physical and neurological exams are necessary and can be accomplished in a short period of time if a methodical approach is used. The physical examination of the headache patient should include a general examination of the lungs, heart, and abdomen, as well as a detailed examination of the scalp and neck (Box 9.3). Repeatedly using the same sequence of examination tests in each patient results in an efficient and complete evaluation. Blood work may be indicated in patients with symptoms or signs suggesting specific medical illnesses and in patients >50 years old (e.g., to rule out giant cell or temporal arteritis).

Box 9.3 Evaluation of new-onset or worrisome headaches (Adapted from Marcus DA. Chronic pain. A primary care guide to practical management. 2nd edition, Humana Press, Totowa, NJ, 2008.)

- History and physical examination
  - Complete review of systems
  - Vital signs (including weight, temperature, blood pressure, heart rate, and respirations)
  - Cervical spine examination
    - Resting posture in a normal or forward position
    - Active range of motion for decreased movement or crepitance
    - Palpation for localized tenderness
  - Neurological evaluation
    - Gait
    - Fundoscopy for papilledema[a]
    - Assess symmetry of face and eye movements
    - Strength and reflex testing

- ■ Sensation to touch
- ■ Able to identify 2 of 3 numbers drawn in the palm without looking

- Laboratory
  - Radiological testing

    - ■ Computed tomography or magnetic resonance imaging (MRI) of brain if red flags present/secondary headache is suspected and testing will change treatment recommendations
    - ■ X-ray cervical spine for mechanical abnormalities[b] if testing will change treatment recommendations
    - ■ MRI of cervical spine for radiculopathy[c] if testing will change treatment recommendations

  - Lab work when medical history or examination suggests general medical illness

    - ■ Autoimmune tests (antinuclear antibody), though rarely helpful as frequent false positives
    - ■ Hematology (blood count)

        - ➢ Sedimentation rate/C-reactive protein and temporal arteritis workup for new headache in patients aged >50 years
        - ➢ Anemia, low platelets in pre-eclampsia/eclampsia

    - ■ Chemistries (electrolytes; liver and kidney function tests)
    - ■ Urinalysis for proteinuria in pre-eclampsia/eclampsia
    - ■ Endocrine (thyroid function tests)
    - ■ Infectious (rapid plasma reagin for syphilis, HIV testing)

[a]Fundoscopic examination may be enhanced by using the Welch Allyn Panoptic fundoscope, which provides a magnified view for easier viewing. (Details available at http://www.welchallyn.com/promotions/PanOptic).
[b]Mechanical abnormalities include abnormal posture, restricted range of motion, or pain reproduced with neck motion.
[c]Radiculopathy should be considered if focal strength, reflex, or sensory loss in an arm is present.

Specialized testing (including a spinal fluid examination and neuroimaging) may be indicated in patients whose histories or examinations suggest secondary causes of headache, such as meningitis, brain tumors, subarachnoid hemorrhage, or intracranial aneurysms. Radiographic imaging of the cervical spine is typically delayed until after delivery, unless treatment will be altered based on results during pregnancy.

Spinal Fluid Examination

A lumbar puncture is important in cases of suspected inflammatory disease (such as meningitis), subarachnoid hemorrhage, or benign intracranial hypertension. As in non-pregnant patients, an imaging study of the head should be performed prior to lumbar puncture when:

- Headache began after trauma;
- Increased intracranial pressure or hemorrhage is suspected;
- Seizure has occurred;
- Patient has altered level of consciousness or focal neurological signs.

Spinal fluid examinations can be safely performed and easily interpreted during pregnancy, with appearance, opening pressure, cell count, and protein levels similar between non-pregnant and pregnant women [3]. A comparison of spinal fluid examinations in women who had spinal anesthesia performed for delivery ($N = 44$) or tubal ligation ($N = 22$) showed no differences in opening pressure, cell count, or protein levels between patient groups [3]. In addition, spinal fluid results were unaffected by active labor, length of gestation, and type of delivery (vaginal versus Cesarean section). Therefore, abnormal values obtained during pregnancy should not be attributed to the pregnancy itself, but must be further evaluated as in the non-pregnant patient.

As in non-pregnant or lactating patients, the spinal fluid examination for headache during pregnancy or when nursing should include assessments of opening pressure, fluid appearance, cell count, protein, and glucose. Headache may occur in patients with elevated pressures, such as benign intracranial hypertension, or low pressures, such as low pressure post-spinal anesthesia. Cytology should be evaluated in patients with a history of malignancy. Additional testing for infectious conditions will also be needed in

Table 9.1 Normal adult lumbar puncture results (Based on [4])

Test	Normal value
Appearance	Clear and colorless
Opening pressure in lateral recumbent position	180 mm H_2O (200–250 mm H_2O in obese patient)
White blood cells	0–5 mononuclear cells (lymphocytes and monocytes) 0 polymorphonuclear leukocytes
Glucose	65% of serum glucose <45 mg/dL is abnormal
Protein	≤50 mg/dL

immuno-compromised or immune-suppressed patients. Expected normal lumbar puncture results are given in Table 9.1 [4].

> ***Pearl for the practitioner:***
> Spinal fluid examination during pregnancy should produce similar normal results to those seen in non-pregnant women. Abnormal spinal fluid results should not be attributed to pregnancy.

Neuroimaging

In general, neuroimaging studies are not recommended for any patient with chronic headache unless she develops a new headache pattern or abnormal neurological signs or symptoms, such as focal abnormalities, mental status changes, or seizures [5]. Abnormalities on magnetic resonance imaging (MRI) scans are expected to be present in a significant minority of headache sufferers [6]. The most common abnormalities are nonspecific white matter changes, which occur in about 30% of migraine patients. The etiology and significance of these white matter changes are uncertain.

Neuroimaging is often necessary in patients with a change in headache pattern, with or without evidence of focal neurological abnormalities. Imaging studies should be considered when the patient's history or examination suggests neurological conditions for which an imaging study will potentially alter treatment during pregnancy (Box 9.4). In both pregnant and non-pregnant patients, MRI is preferred over computed tomography (CT) when brain imaging is recommended for non-emergent or non-traumatic headache. MRI provides a clearer picture of soft tissues and brain structures, while CT better clarifies hemorrhage and fractures. CT imaging, therefore, is generally preferred in patients with headache following acute trauma or when intracranial bleeding is suspected.

Pearl for the practitioner:
MRI is the preferred neuroimaging study for patients with non-traumatic headache. CT is preferred after trauma or when intracranial hemorrhage is suspected.

Box 9.4 Differential diagnoses in pregnant headache patients suggesting consideration for neuroimaging and/or other testing

- Benign intracranial hypertension (pseudotumor cerebri)—lumbar puncture
- Central venous thrombosis—MR venogram
- Cerebrovascular accident (hemorrhagic or thrombotic)—MRI
- Eclampsia with neurological complications—urinalysis, hematology
- Metastatic disease (e.g., patients with breast cancer, melanoma, or choriocarcinoma)—MRI
- Subarachnoid hemorrhage/possible intracranial aneurysm—CT scan, MR angiogram
- Trauma (e.g., with subdural hematoma)—CT
- Tumor (e.g., pituitary adenoma or meningioma)—MRI
- Vasculitis (e.g., in patients with systemic lupus erythematosus)—MRI, autoimmune tests, hematology, urinalysis

CT = computed tomography, MR = magnetic resonance, MRI = magnetic resonance imaging

In a retrospective review of 63 pregnant women reporting to an emergency department for a primary complaint of headache, MRI or CT studies were normal or revealed only incidental/nonspecific findings in most of these women (73%) [7]. Pathological conditions included sinusitis (8%), cerebral venous thrombosis (6%), reversible posterior leukoencephalopathy/eclampsia (6%), benign intracranial hypertension (pseudotumor cerebri) (3%), and intracranial hemorrhage (3%). Among patients with abnormal neurological examinations, a pathological condition was identified in 38% of patients. Among patients with normal neurological examinations, a pathological scan occurred in 19% of patients. Therefore, although the presence of an abnormal neurological exam predicts increased likelihood of intracranial pathology, absence of an abnormal examination alone does not provide adequate assurance of no intracranial pathology.

Pearl for the practitioner:
A normal neurological examination alone is not sensitive enough to exclude intracranial pathology. Neuroimaging may still be indicated even if the neurological exam is normal.

Computed Tomography

Although radiation is preferably avoided during pregnancy, CT imaging may be necessary in some women with head trauma, abnormal neurological examinations, or headaches suggesting intracranial hemorrhage. CT should be utilized in those cases where it is considered medically necessary and the results will potentially change treatment during pregnancy. Fetal effects depend on both the timing and dosage of radiation exposure (Table 9.2) [8]. In general, fetal radiation exposure from a maternal head CT is well below levels that have been linked to fetal effects (Table 9.3) [9–11]. Fetal exposure to ionizing radiation from a maternal head CT is extremely low (<0.005 mGy) and considered to be substantially less risky for the fetus than not identifying and treating potentially serious neurological conditions in the mother [12]. In a recent paper, the safety of maternal head CT was further supported by arguing that, while the risk of childhood leukemia was increased after exposure to 1–2 rads in utero, the average head CT results in an estimated fetal radiation dose of <0.01 rad [13]. (For conversion, 1 rad = 10 mGy). Fetal exposure from a maternal head CT results from scatter throughout the body rather than directed radiation. Therefore, abdominal shielding will do little to reduce fetal radiation exposure from a head CT, although it may reduce maternal anxiety.

Table 9.2 Teratogenic effects of radiation exposure (Based on [8])

Weeks gestation	Developmental stage	Fetal effects	Radiation dose threshold (mGy)
0–2	Pre-implantation	No effect or death	50–100
2–8	Organogenesis	Malformations Growth retardation	200
8–15	Early fetal development	Mental retardation	60–310
16–25	Later fetal development	Mental retardation	250–280

Table 9.3 Typical radiation doses (Based on [9,10,11])

	Rad	mGy
Fetal exposure from cervical spine x-ray	<1 rad	<0.001 mGy
Fetal exposure from maternal head CT	<1 rad	<0.005 mGy
Safe fetal dose	<5 rads	<50 mGy
Doses with fetal effects	20–40 rads between 8 and 15 weeks gestation increases risk for mental retardation	300–1000 mGy increases risks for failure to implant, abortion, growth retardation, central nervous system effects

> **Pearl for the practitioner:**
> Fetal exposure to ionizing radiation from a maternal head CT is extremely low and considered to be substantially less risky for the fetus than an undiagnosed, potentially serious intracranial condition in the mother.

Magnetic Resonance Imaging

Magnetic resonance imaging (MRI) is preferred over traditional radiographic testing during pregnancy. MRI exposure during pregnancy is generally considered to be safe [14], with no negative sequelae identified during evaluations of three-year-olds exposed to MRI in utero [15] or the offspring of female MRI technicians [16]. Currently, the American College of Radiology recommends MRI during pregnancy to avoid exposure to ionizing radiation when imaging studies are needed and the results of testing may change patient care [17]. Furthermore, cerebral vasculature may be effectively visualized using non-invasive MRI angiography or venography.

> **Pearl for the practitioner:**
> MRI is the preferred brain imaging modality, if necessary, in pregnant women because of its lack of ionizing radiation.

Contrast Agents During Pregnancy

The 11th European Symposium on Urogenital Radiology conducted an extensive literature review of the use of iodinated and gadolinium contrast during pregnancy and lactation [18]. Recommendations are given in Table 9.4. In general, contrast agents may be used during pregnancy

Table 9.4 Recommendations for using contrast agents (Based on [18])

Contrast agent	Pregnancy	Lactation
Iodinated contrast	Use when necessary information will be gathered from imaging study. Contrast improves identification of tumors and abscesses. Screen newborn for thyroid function.	Safe to continue nursing after exposure
Gadolinium contrast	Use when necessary information will be gathered from imaging study. Contrast improves identification of tumors and abscesses.	Safe to continue nursing after exposure

when they are deemed necessary [18]. Contrast agents are particularly helpful in identifying secondary causes of headache, such as neoplasms and abscesses, that may be missed on a non-contrasted study. Maternal exposure to iodinated contrast agents during pregnancy can depress fetal and neonatal thyroid function. The fetal thyroid begins synthesizing thyroxine (T4) by 12 weeks of gestation and triiodothyronine (T3) after 30 weeks. In general, infants are screened for hypothyroidism during their first week of life, with this screening particularly imperative in babies exposed to in utero iodinated contrast. Fortunately, no fetal effects have been documented from intrauterine gadolinium exposure.

> ***Pearl for the practitioner:***
> Iodinated contrast imaging (e.g., CT with contrast) can depress neonatal thyroid function. MRI is preferred over CT with contrast. If CT with contrast is necessary, thyroid function in the neonate should be checked in the first postpartum week. Contrast with MRI (i.e., gadolinium) is considered to be safe for the developing baby.

Contrast Agents During Lactation

Only small amounts of iodinated or gadolinium contrast agents are expected in breast milk [18]. For example, a study testing gadolinium excretion into breast milk in 20 lactating women showed that <0.04% of the administered dose was excreted into the breast milk, which is over 100 times below the permitted neonatal intravenous dosage [19]. Consequently, the 11th European Symposium on Urogenital Radiology recommended no temporary cessation of breastfeeding when contrast agents are used in lactating women [18]. This recommendation to continue to nurse after exposure to contrast agents has been supported by others, who argue that temporarily discontinuing breastfeeding is not scientifically indicated and may result in undesirable exposure for the baby to nonphysiological formula, introduction of foreign proteins, and subsequent problems with nursing or refusal to breastfeed [20].

Summary

The general principles guiding headache evaluation in non-pregnant patients similarly apply during pregnancy and lactation. A detailed history is the most important diagnostic tool in headache patients. All patients will additionally require a complete medical evaluation and neurological screening. Specialized testing is guided by the differential diagnosis; however, spinal fluid examinations and neuroimaging should be performed in patients for whom the testing is necessary and the results will potentially modify treatment.

Practical pointers:

- Most headaches in pregnant women are primary headaches, usually migraine and tension-type. Secondary headaches are rare, but potentially ominous and should be considered.
- A thorough history is essential when evaluating headache. Questions should target identifying possible alarm symptoms/red flags.
- Focused physical and neurological exams can be performed efficiently, especially if a consistent, methodical approach is used.
- Spinal fluid examination may be indicated in cases of suspected infection, inflammation, subarachnoid hemorrhage, or benign intracranial hypertension. Normal spinal fluid findings are similar in pregnant and non-pregnant women.
- If brain imaging is necessary, MRI is the preferred test as it does not use ionizing radiation. CT may be preferred in cases of trauma or suspected hemorrhage.
- Contrast agents, if necessary, may be used when pregnant or breast-feeding. Iodinated agents used with CT scanning can depress fetal thyroid and thus, if used, require thyroid testing of the newborn during the first week of life.

References

1. Ertresvg JM, Stovner LJ, Kvavik LE, et al. Migraine aura or transient ischemic attacks? A five-year follow-up case-controlled study of women with transient central nervous system disorders in pregnancy. *BMC Medicine* 2007;5:19.
2. Ramirez-Lassepas M, Espinosa CE, Cicero JJ, et al. Predictors of intracranial pathological findings in patients who seek emergency care because of headache. *Arch Neurol* 1997;54:1506–1509.
3. Davis LE. Normal laboratory values of CSF during pregnancy. *Arch Neurol* 1979;36:443.
4. Roos KL. Lumbar puncture. *Semin Neurol* 2003;23:105–114.
5. Sandrini G, Friberg L, Jänig W, et al. Neurophysiological tests and neuroimaging procedures in non-acute headache: guidelines and recommendations. *Eur J Neurol* 2004;11:217–224.
6. Marcus DA. Central nervous system abnormalities in migraine. *Expert Opin Pharmacother* 2003;4:1709–1715.
7. Ramchandren S, Cross BJ, Liebeskind DS. Emergent headaches during pregnancy: correlation between neurologic examination and neuroimaging. *Am J Neuroradiol* 2007;28:1085–1087.
8. Patel SJ, Reede DL, Katz DS, Subramaniam R, Amorosa JK. Imaging the pregnant patient for nonobstetric conditions: algorithms and radiation dose considerations. *Radiography* 2007;27:1705–1722.
9. American College of Obstetricians and Gynaecologists Committee Opinion. Guidelines for diagnostic imaging during pregnancy. *Obstet Gynecol* 2004;104:647–651.

10. Lowe SA. Diagnostic radiography in pregnancy: risks and reality. *Aust N Z J Obstet Gynaecol* 2004;44:191–196.
11. McCollough CH, Schueler BA, Atwell TD, et al. Radiation exposure and pregnancy: when should we be concerned? *Radiographics* 2007;27:909–918.
12. Dineen R, Banks A, Lenthall R. Imaging of acute neurological conditions in pregnancy and the puerperium. *Clin Radiol* 2005;60:1156–1170.
13. Brass SD, Copen WA. Neurological disorders in pregnancy from a neuroimaging perspective. *Semin Neurol* 2007;5:411–424.
14. Levine D, Barnes PD, Edleman RR. Obstetric MR imaging. *Radiology* 1999;211:609–617.
15. Baker P, Johnson I, Harvey P, Mansfield P. A three-year follow-up of children imaged in utero using echo-planar magnetic resonance. *Am J Obstet Gynecol* 1994;170:32–33.
16. Kanal E, Gillen J, Evans J, Savitz D, Shellock F. Survey of reproductive health among female MR workers. *Radiology* 1993;187:395–399.
17. ACR standards: MRI safety and sedation. Available at http://acr.org. Accessed March 2008.
18. Webb JW, Thomsen HS, Morcos SK. The use of iodinated and gadolinium contrast media during pregnancy and lactation. *Eur Radiol* 2005;15:1234–1240.
19. Kubik-Huch RA, Gottstein-Aalame NM, Frenzel T, et al. Gadopentatate dimeglumine excretion into human breast milk during lactation. *Radiology* 2000;216:555–558.
20. Newman J. Breastfeeding and radiologic procedures. *Can Fam Physician* 2007;53: 630–631.

Chapter 10
Patient Headache Resources

Key Chapter Points

- Patients who have recurrent headaches are usually very eager to learn as much as they can about their headache condition.
- Patient education can empower patients to participate more fully in their headache care.
- Patient education is an often overlooked facet of good headache care.
- Many well done, easy-to-read patient educational materials are available covering a wide variety of headache topics.
- This chapter provides practical patient handouts and resources that can be used in a busy clinical practice. A CD-ROM accompanies this book that contains the patient handouts, allowing for easy reprinting.

Keywords Education· Exercise· Handout· Reference· Relaxation· Training

Educating patients is an essential, though often overlooked, component of effective headache management. In an interesting survey, both headache doctors and headache patients were asked about important aspects of care [1]. Education was the top priority for patients, but was considered important by only a minority of doctors. Additionally, 86% of the patients rated the receipt of answers to their questions as important compared with only 15% of doctors. Similarly, educating patients about headaches and teaching patients how to treat attacks were rated important by 72% of patients and only 15% of doctors. Although patients understand the importance of education, clinicians have only recently realized the valuable therapeutic value that education has in the comprehensive care of headache patients. Educated patients usually feel more empowered to take a more active role in the treatment of their headaches.

> ***Pearl for the practitioner:***
> Patients with recurring headaches are often eager to learn as much as they can about their headache condition.

D.A. Marcus, P.A. Bain, *Effective Migraine Treatment in Pregnant
and Lactating Women: A Practical Guide*, DOI 10.1007/978-1-60327-439-5_10,
© Humana Press, a part of Springer Science+Business Media, LLC 2009

Unfortunately, adequately educating headache patients during a busy office visit can sometimes be challenging. Many issues often have to be covered in the brief time allotted for an office visit. Take-home handouts can provide valuable information to supplement and reinforce education received during office visits. Materials can be provided to explain treatment recommendations and promote specific skill training. Routinely incorporating written materials into headache visits can substantially improve headache care. For example, patients provided with self-administered educational materials for learning pain management skills for home use experienced considerable reductions in headache frequency and disability (Fig. 10.1) [2].

> *Pearl for the practitioner:*
> Providing patient education materials and resources is an effective, time efficient component of good headache care.

This chapter contains a wide variety of patient handouts and educational materials that can be reproduced and given to patients. A CD-ROM accompanies this book that contains these handouts, allowing for easy downloading and printing. Here is a listing of the handouts available in this chapter:

- General information
  - When you're ready to get pregnant
    - Important proactive treatment recommendations before conception
  - Now that you're pregnant
    - Various headache treatment options during pregnancy and lactation
  - After you've delivered
    - Effective treatment options that can be used when nursing
  - Daily headache diary
    - Weekly headache and treatment recording log to assist with identifying headache and medication use patterns and response to treatment

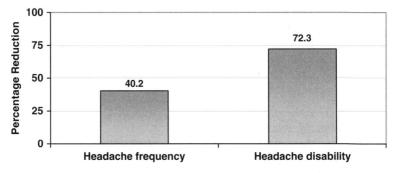

Fig. 10.1 Benefits of self-administered psychological pain management (Based on [2])

- Headache treatment
  - Now that I'm trying to get pregnant, what can I do when I get a headache?
    - Stratified approach to safe acute headache treatment during pregnancy.
  - What non-drug treatments are effective for treating headaches?
    - Broad overview of the wide range of effective non-drug treatments
  - Practicing relaxation techniques
    - Instruction on using a variety of relaxation techniques
  - Stress management
    - Introduction to stress management
  - Headache-reducing exercises
    - Instructional guide for aerobic and stretching exercises

- Nausea treatment
  - What can I do if I'm feeling nauseated during my pregnancy?
    - Dietary tips to help reduce pregnancy-related nausea

- Additional headache resources
  - Where can I find reliable online information about migraine and other headaches?
    - List of useful Internet headache resources, including resources useful for pregnant and breastfeeding patients
  - Where can I learn more about managing my headaches?
    - List of books and other resources for managing headaches

Patient handouts are not designed to replace good communication with the healthcare provider; however, these sheets can reinforce and supplement those messages provided during a visit. In addition, providing written materials also increases both the clarity and the credibility of recommendations, and saves time during an already full clinic visit.

References

1. Lipton RB, Stewart WF. Acute migraine therapy: do doctors understand what patients with migraine want from therapy? *Headache* 1999;39(Suppl 2):S20–S26.
2. Nicholson R, Nash J, Andrasik F. A self-administered behavioral intervention using tailored messages for migraine. *Headache* 2005;45:1124–1139.

General Information

When you're ready to get pregnant ...

Congratulations on your decision to have a baby. The best time to prepare for your pregnancy is before you become pregnant. This is the ideal time to make decisions about safer headache treatments.

The good news is that most women experience headache improvement with pregnancy:

- Headaches improve for about four in every five women by the third trimester.
- Headaches often don't improve until the early second trimester.
- Even if your headaches improve, you may still continue to have some troublesome headaches that will need treatment.
- Safer and effective treatments are available when trying to get pregnant and after you have become pregnant.

Before you start trying to get pregnant, you should talk to your doctor about your headache treatment. You will need to:

- Learn safe and effective non-drug treatments that you can use to control headaches throughout your pregnancy and after delivery.
- Make sure the headache medications you are using are safe for you to take when trying to get pregnant and throughout pregnancy. This reduces risks to the baby if you become pregnant while taking the medications.
- Try to get your headache pattern under as good control as possible before becoming pregnant.
- Talk to your doctor before using any non-prescription medications and supplements to make sure they are safe during pregnancy.

Often, medication choices need to change with pregnancy to make sure you minimize risks to your baby.

Remember, there are many safer and effective non-drug and drug treatments for you to use throughout your pregnancy. Making treatment changes before you become pregnant is the best way to provide the safest treatments for your developing baby.

Now that you're pregnant ...

Congratulations on becoming pregnant!

As soon as you know that you're pregnant, make an appointment to talk to your doctor about your headaches. You will need to learn:

- Safe and effective non-drug treatments to control your headaches;
- Which medications you can safely take for pain and nausea;
- Which medications you can safely take to prevent headaches if this becomes necessary;
- What to do if your headaches get worse.

Let your doctor know:

- What your current headache pattern is like;
- If there has been any recent change in your headaches;
- If you are having any other medical problems besides headaches;
- What over-the-counter medications you are taking;
- What supplements, vitamins, minerals, and herbs you are taking;
- What prescription medications you are taking and who prescribed them.

Know that you are not expected to suffer with your headaches during pregnancy. Headaches improve for four in every five women, so the odds are good that your headaches will get better.

General recommendations for pregnant patients who have headaches:

- Quit smoking.
- Eat regular meals and snacks—don't skip meals, especially breakfast.
- Get a good night's sleep every night.
- Learn effective relaxation techniques.
- Learn headache-relieving neck stretching exercises.
- Don't use over-the-counter, herbal, or supplement remedies without first discussing them with your healthcare provider.
- Use safe and effective therapies to treat and relieve nausea.
- Develop a plan for treating severe headaches with your doctor. Make sure you know which treatments to try first.
- Talk to your doctor about prevention therapy if you are having frequent severe headaches.

Effectively treating your headaches will allow you to better enjoy your pregnancy.

Even if your headaches aren't a problem during pregnancy, talk to your doctor about safer treatment options that can be used if you decide to breastfeed your baby. Most women experience a return of their previous headaches after delivery. Fortunately, breastfeeding often delays the return of headaches. There are more headache treatment options available when you're breastfeeding compared to during pregnancy. Some medications should be avoided during breastfeeding. Work with your provider to develop a safe, effective treatment plan.

After you've delivered ...

Congratulations on your new arrival! An exciting new chapter in your life has begun!

While four out of five women note improvement in their headache pattern by the third trimester, headaches usually return after delivery. Headaches may return after your baby is born because of changes in:

- Hormone levels;
- Your sleep pattern;
- Stress associated with the new arrival and changing routines.

All of these factors can contribute to the return of the headaches.

After your baby is born, your headaches can affect both you and your ability to interact with your baby—so there are now even more reasons to effectively control your headaches. Medications you use for your headaches can also affect the baby if you are nursing, so talk to your healthcare provider about which medications can be safely used when nursing. Fortunately, many effective headache treatments can be used while breastfeeding.

The decision to breastfeed your infant is an important one. There are many health benefits for the breastfed newborn, as well as the breastfeeding mother:

- Benefits for the baby from breastfeeding:
  - Ideal nutrition;
  - Gives baby important hormones and immune factors;
  - Reduces infant infections;
  - Promotes bonding with mom.

- Benefits for the mother from breastfeeding:
  - Delays return of headaches;
  - Helps improve needed weight loss after delivery;
  - Reduces the risk for developing breast and ovarian cancer;
  - Reduces the risk for developing rheumatoid arthritis;
  - Promotes bonding with baby.

If you decide to nurse your baby:

- Arrange an office visit with your healthcare provider soon after delivery to develop a safe, effective treatment plan.
- Review non-drug approaches to treat headaches.
- Keep track of your headaches using a headache diary.
- Learn how and when to safely store breast milk in case you need to supplement feedings.
- Talk to your provider about safe and effective contraceptive methods that can be used when breastfeeding.

Daily Headache Diary

Name: _____ First day of diary (Sunday) ____/____/_____

Day	Migraine Severity				Treatments	
	None	Mild	Moderate	Severe	Medications	Non-medications
Sunday						
Morning						
Noon						
Evening						
Bedtime						
Monday						
Morning						
Noon						
Evening						
Bedtime						
Tuesday						
Morning						
Noon						
Evening						
Bedtime						
Wednesday						
Morning						
Noon						
Evening						
Bedtime						
Thursday						
Morning						
Noon						
Evening						
Bedtime						
Friday						
Morning						
Noon						
Evening						
Bedtime						
Saturday						
Morning						
Noon						
Evening						
Bedtime						

Instructions: record headache severity every day, four times daily. Also record all treatment you used each day.

Headache Treatment

Now that I'm trying to get pregnant, what can I do when I get a headache?

Acute migraine medications are used to treat severe migraine episodes. Regularly using acute medications more than two days per week can worsen your headaches and result in medication overuse or rebound headaches. Let your doctor know if you are using or need to use acute medication more than two days per week.

When you get a migraine, remember the following principles:

- Start with non-drug treatments.
- Don't take medication for mild headaches.
  - When you take a medication, use only medications recommended by your doctor and use the recommended dose.
- If nausea occurs with your migraine, ask your doctor for recommendations to treat and reduce nausea.

When you get a mild migraine:

- Apply heat or ice (whichever you find more soothing) for 20 minutes to your temples or neck.
- Begin relaxation techniques: deep breathing, imagery, or biofeedback.
- Use acupressure techniques (described in *What non-drug treatments are effective for treating headaches?* handout).
- Include positive messages about good expectations.
- Do oscillatory movements (described in *Headache-reducing exercises* handout).
- Perform exercises that stretch your painful area. Be sure to stretch slowly, and only to the point of first feeling a stretching sensation.
- Use distraction techniques.
- Don't give up—combining and repeating these techniques is usually helpful.

When you get a moderate migraine:

- Use those techniques for mild migraine.
- If non-drug treatments haven't worked, use acetaminophen.
- Treat nausea with non-drug therapies and, if necessary, medications (See *What can I do if I'm feeling nauseated during my pregnancy* handout.)

When you get a severe migraine:

- Use the tools for mild plus moderate migraine.
- If acetaminophen and non-drug treatments haven't worked, talk to your doctor about other treatments, such as benadryl, lidocaine nasal spray, or a mild narcotic.
- If possible, going to sleep can turn off a severe migraine.

Keep track of your headaches in diaries and bring completed diaries to your next visit to see how well your treatment is working. Mark when you get a headache, how bad it was on a 1–10 scale, whether you had significant nausea with it, and how well your treatments worked.

Do not use any additional over-the-counter, supplement, or prescription drugs without first talking with your healthcare provider.

What non-drug treatments are effective for treating headaches?

Non-drug acute headache treatments are designed to block pain messages by sending other signals through the nerves and spinal cord. It's hard for your brain to focus on one thing when it's bombarded with lots of other signals. Pain management techniques are designed to overload brain circuits, blocking transmission of migraine signals. This is similar to having difficulty balancing your checkbook when the television's blaring, the phone is ringing, and toddlers are running through the house. When your brain is occupied with relaxation techniques, moving joints and muscles, or focusing on other activities, it's harder for the brain to have enough excess capacity to also transmit pain messages.

Try to combine several of the following techniques together to maximize the headache relief benefit. Don't be discouraged if these techniques don't always work. Try to use them before your migraine becomes severe. You can also use these in conjunction with doctor-approved migraine medications.

- Apply heat or ice (whichever you find more soothing) for 20 minutes to your temples or neck.
- Begin relaxation techniques: deep breathing, imagery, or biofeedback. Ask your provider if he/she can recommend a local expert who specializes in teaching these techniques.
- Include positive messages about good expectations.
- Do oscillatory movements (described in *Headache-reducing exercises* handout).
- Perform exercises that stretch your painful area. Be sure to stretch slowly, and only to the point of first feeling a stretching sensation.
- Use distraction techniques.
- Try acupuncture.
- If other treatments aren't helping, some people find their headache goes away after a nap. See if sleep can turn off your headache.

Relaxation and biofeedback

- Progressive muscle relaxation involves alternatively contracting and relaxing muscles throughout your body. Close your eyes and practice first tensing and then relaxing individual muscles in different parts of your body, starting at your feet and moving toward your neck and face. Hold the tension for 10–15 seconds, and then release it. Tense and release the muscles in your legs, then abdomen, then arms, then shoulders, then neck, then jaw, then eyes, then forehead. Focus on the sensations of the muscles when they are no longer tensed. When you are familiar with this exercise, you will begin to recognize when your muscles are abnormally tensed, even if you don't feel "stressed." For example, you may notice jaw and neck tension when sitting in traffic or waiting in a line at the store. Once you feel this tension, work to release it.

- Cue-controlled relaxation uses a combination of deep breathing and repetition of the word "relax." Begin this exercise with a slow, deep, abdominal breath. Place your hand over your abdomen to ensure that it is moving in and out with each breath. After inhaling, hold for 5–10 seconds, then exhale, slowly repeating the word "relax." Repeat. After you are comfortable with this technique, you should be able to close your eyes and take a deep breath as above before confronting stressful situations, like a doctor's visit, meeting with the boss, or discussion with your spouse. This will relax your system to reduce the impact of the stressful situations on your pain-provoking physiology and headaches.

Cognitive restructuring

- Replace negative, catastrophic thinking with positive, helpful messages:
  - Instead of thinking, "My day is ruined now," tell yourself, "This migraine will become more manageable soon."
  - Instead of, "Nothing ever gets rid of my migraine," tell yourself, "If I use my acute migraine treatments, the pain will improve soon."
  - Instead of, "Life's not fair. Why me?" remind yourself, "I have good tools to help control my migraine."

Distraction

- Many people suggest lying down in a quiet room when a migraine starts. While this may be necessary when the pain is very severe, you want to try to distract your brain by increasing pleasant stimulation when a migraine starts. When your migraine is still mild-to-moderate, try going for a walk outside, singing to the radio, taking a bike ride, hitting a few golf balls in the backyard, tossing the ball to your dog, or some other pleasurable activity. Avoid activities that are frustrating, require substantial mental exertion, or don't require active engagement (like television viewing).

Heat, ice, and neck stretches

- Apply heat or ice (whichever you find more soothing) for 20 minutes to the neck and shoulders.
- Positional distraction: Place a 1- to 2-inch high stack of books on the floor. Lie on the floor, with the back of your head resting on the books. The edge of the books should be near the middle of your head, so that your neck is free. Relax so that your head moves up from your neck.
- Trigger point compression: You may notice certain spots on your neck muscles that aggravate your pain when you press them. These are called trigger points. Apply pressure to any trigger points with your fingers and hold for 12–60 seconds. Release the pressure, and proceed with your usual stretching exercises. Some physical therapists recommend a Theracane (www.theracane.com) to help apply pressure to hard-to-reach trigger points.
- Oscillatory movements: perform slow, gentle, rhythmic, side-to-side movements of the neck. Face forward and turn your head 1–2 inches, turning

away from the painful side. Return to facing forward. Repeat at a rate of about one turn per second, for a total of 30 seconds. Rest for 30 seconds; then repeat until no further relief is noted. Now turn your head toward the painful side and back, as above.

- Perform neck stretches (described in ***Headache-reducing exercises*** handout).

Acupressure

- Find a depression in the middle of your neck between the neck muscles and move up within this depression to where the neck meets the skull. Rub the area where the neck muscles attach to the skull firmly for 2–3 minutes with deep circular movements.
- Find a depression at each temple, immediately behind your eyebrows. Rub firmly and deeply for 1 minute.
- Find a depression between your eyebrows. Rub firmly and deeply for 1 minute.
- Find the muscle that lies in the web between your thumb and index finger by compressing this area with the thumb and index finger from your other hand. Deeply and firmly make circular motions over this area for 5 minutes. Repeat with your other hand.

Sleep

- Going to bed with a migraine should be reserved for severe episodes associated with nausea that prevents physical activity.
- Sleep can effectively shut off serotonin-activated pain pathways. Some people find a 1-hour nap effectively relieves their migraine. Unless your headache is severe, avoid bed unless you also experience fairly prompt headache relief from brief sleep.

Practicing relaxation techniques

Relaxation techniques are very effective for controlling chronic headaches. These techniques have been shown to be very effective during pregnancy and while nursing. Interestingly, headache reduction from relaxation techniques is just as good as that from typical headache medications. The good news is you don't have to worry about medication exposure with relaxation.

You may be planning to learn breathing techniques, like Lamaze, to help control your pain when your baby is delivered. You will learn these skills months before you will actually use them to control pain at the time of delivery. No one can learn these techniques once they're in the middle of having contractions. Similarly, you have to first practice headache-relieving relaxation techniques when you don't have a bad headache. You should practice these skills several times daily until you feel you have developed a good ability to achieve a relaxed state. Then you can use them effectively to help control headache pain when a headache first begins.

Relaxation techniques work by getting your brain to turn on pain-relieving centers. Relaxation techniques release the same brain chemicals that control headaches when you take headache medications. This is why these techniques are so helpful. So it's not a matter of "chilling out" or "letting things roll off of your back." Relaxation techniques are really a way to tap into your body's natural pain-relieving pathways.

Tips for performing relaxation techniques

- Relaxation techniques should be learned while sitting in a comfortable chair, with arms and legs uncrossed, feet flat on the floor, and eyes closed.
- Each practice session should last for about 15–20 uninterrupted minutes.
- Once you have regularly practiced and mastered these techniques, you will be able to use them whenever you feel yourself starting to tense or in anticipation of stress.
- Several effective techniques are progressive muscle relaxation, cue-controlled relaxation, and thermal biofeedback. Each is described below.

Progressive muscle relaxation

Progressive muscle relaxation involves alternately contracting and relaxing muscles throughout your body.

- Close your eyes and practice first tensing and then relaxing individual muscles in different parts of your body, starting at your feet and moving toward your neck and face.
- Hold the tension for 10–15 seconds, and then release it.
- Tense and release the muscles in your legs, then abdomen, then arms, then shoulders, then neck, then jaw, then eyes, then forehead.
- Focus on how the muscles feel when they are no longer tensed.

- When you are familiar with this exercise, you will begin to recognize when your muscles are unusually tense, even if you don't feel "stressed." For example, you may notice jaw and neck tightness when sitting in traffic or waiting in a line at the store. Once you feel this tightness, work to relax it as you do during your quiet training sessions.

Cue-controlled relaxation

Cue-controlled relaxation uses a combination of deep breathing and repetition of the word "relax."

- Begin this exercise with a slow, deep, abdominal breath.
- Place your hand over your abdomen to make sure that it is moving in and out with each breath. After breathing in, hold your breath for 5–10 seconds, then breathe out, slowly repeating the word "relax." Repeat.
- After you are comfortable with this method, you should be able to close your eyes and take a deep breath as above before dealing with stressful situations, like a doctor's visit, a meeting with the boss, or a discussion with your spouse. This will relax your system and reduce the effect of the stressful situation on your pain-provoking mechanisms and headaches.

Thermal biofeedback

Place a handheld thermometer on your finger and measure the temperature.

- Focus on raising your finger temperature by 2–3 degrees Fahrenheit (probably to about 96 degrees) while practicing relaxation techniques.
- Some people find that it's difficult to "feel" relaxed. Using biofeedback can help show you when you are getting relaxed. If you are turning on and turning off the right pathways in your brain and nervous system, this will result in a feeling of calm, higher skin temperatures, and, most importantly, the blocking of pain messages.
- An inexpensive finger thermometer and biofeedback audiotape may be obtained from Primary Care Network (1-800-769-7565).

Stress management

Stress is consistently reported as the #1 trigger for both migraine and tension-type headaches, acting as a trigger for about 75% of headache sufferers. Remember that everyone experiences stress symptoms, with our bodies reacting in different ways to stress. Some people become loud and boisterous, others quiet and reserved. Other people experience chest pain, rapid breathing, stomach aches, or diarrhea. Typically, people notice that stress causes their usual health symptoms to be aggravated. Stress can cause people with heart disease to experience chest pain, people with Parkinson's disease more tremors, people with epilepsy a higher risk of seizures, and headache sufferers headaches.

Stress management does not mean ignoring or eliminating stressful situations from our lives. Indeed, every life is full of stresses related to school, work, family, health issues, etc. In fact, driving to your doctor's office may be stressful because of traffic and concerns about making it to the appointment on time. Your doctor would not suggest that you "eliminate" the stress of your appointment. And no one could imagine that having a new baby in the house won't be stressful!

While it is not usually possible to change whatever is producing the stress response, we can change our response to the stress. Stress management teaches your body to react to stresses in different ways that do not result in the release of pain-provoking chemicals and tightening muscles. So, when you're stuck in aggravating city traffic on your way to your appointment, instead of experiencing a flare in temper, clenching your teeth, and tightening the muscles in your neck, you can repeat soothing thoughts ("I will make my appointment. I am a responsible person.") or listen to music, while practicing relaxation techniques (such as slow, deep breathing). These same strategies can be used before attending a meeting with one's boss or a child's teacher, before beginning a discussion about family issues with your spouse or child, or when waiting in a long line at the grocery store.

Try these stress management techniques:

- Learn good time management: schedule a reasonable amount of activities, chores, or goals for each day. Overloading your schedule will inevitably result in a stress response.
  - Write down which activities must be completed each day, and delegate chores among members of your household.
  - Accept that life won't be perfect. It's more important to have a relaxed home than a spotless house.
  - Don't be afraid to say no. You can't volunteer for every worthwhile cause and your kids don't need to participate in every possible after-school activity. Prioritize what's important for you and your family.
  - Schedule down time every day for reading, reflection, or a fun family activity.

- Identify your stress buttons. Learn what events typically make you feel stressed. You might be stressed after meeting with your boss, helping with a school project, or talking with your mother-in-law.
  - Anticipate when your stress buttons will be pushed, and practice relaxation techniques beforehand.
  - Stretch muscles when they first become tense.
  - Provide positive encouraging messages to yourself before the beginning of a stressful activity to reduce your stress response.

- Practice daily stress-busting:
  - Recognize and accept stressful events you can't control (e.g., the weather or other people's attitudes and behavior).
  - Plan for stress by recognizing when stressful events are likely to occur.
  - Practice relaxation techniques and cognitive restructuring.
  - Ask for help from others—you don't have to do everything yourself!
  - Do aerobic exercise every day.
  - Consider learning and practicing yoga, Tai Chi, and/or mindfulness meditation.
  - Eat regularly.
  - Get plenty of sleep.
  - Sing and find humor in your day.

Most people notice stress symptoms when they come upon new environments and situations. Take time to spot situations that are usually stress-provoking for you. When you feel your jaw or hands clench or notice you are beginning to sweat before certain situations, make a mental note that these events are stressful for you. For some people, events like taking a test in school or giving a speech or a business presentation may be where they feel stress. For others, minor events, like making a phone call, driving in traffic, or meeting a school teacher may be stress-provoking. Understanding your body's response to stress lets you understand how and when to best use relaxation techniques and stress management.

Headache-reducing exercises

Helpful exercises for headache typically include both aerobic and stretching exercises.

Aerobic exercise

In general, low–impact physical activity and exercise should be maintained during uncomplicated pregnancies. Aerobic exercises are typically performed daily, beginning at a low level, then increasing as tolerated. Walking, swimming, and bicycling are all good aerobic exercises. A walking program often begins at about $\frac{1}{8}$ to $\frac{1}{4}$ mile per day, increased by $\frac{1}{8}$ to $\frac{1}{4}$ mile each week until achieving a target of 1–2 miles per day. You should always discuss plans for any exercise program with your obstetrician. In general, low–impact activities performed routinely before pregnancy can be continued.

Stretching exercises

Stretching exercises should be relaxing. They should be done daily, with each session lasting about 25 minutes. Stretches should result in a normal sensation of stretching, but not pain. Hold the stretch for 5 seconds, relax for 5–10 seconds, and then repeat each stretch about 3–5 times.

Several specific exercises are described below. You may perform several repetitions of each exercise during every exercise session, or vary stretches between exercise sessions.

- Neck range of motion: bend your chin to your chest, then rotate chin to each shoulder, then tip your ear toward your shoulder, then pull in your chin to make a double chin.
- Shoulder shrugs: sit/stand up straight and raise your shoulders straight up. Lower and relax. Then raise shoulders up and forward. Lower and relax. Then raise shoulders up and back.
- Suboccipital range of motion: place a rolled or folded towel behind your neck and gently pull down. Tilt your chin to your chest. Look up at the ceiling. Tilt your ear toward your shoulder.
- Neck stretches: tilt your ear to the shoulder on the same side. Then tilt your chin forward and toward the opposite breast. Gently press with your hand at the end of the stretch to feel the stretch.
- Neck isometrics: place your palm on your forehead and press your head against it, keeping your palm stationary. Don't let your head or hand move. Repeat with your hand on each side of your head.
- Head lift: place folded hands behind your neck at the base of your head. Pull elbows forward and up to achieve the sensation of lifting the head up slightly from the neck.
- Turtle: with head looking forward, push the chin forward, away from the neck. When the head is forward, turn about 1 inch to each side and up.

Schedule twice-daily stretching sessions, each lasting about 15 minutes. Stretching in the morning and before bed can help relieve stress before starting the day and aid with relaxation before sleep. Alternatively, you might include stretching exercises when watching your favorite daily television programs.

The stretching exercises that are particularly soothing for you can also be performed when you feel the beginning of a headache or muscle tension throughout the day. Many stretching exercises can be performed while standing or sitting and can act as stress-releasers when sitting in a long meeting or in the car, waiting in line at the store, or standing in the shower.

Acute headache relief techniques

Acute headache relief techniques can be used when a headache has already occurred, to help minimize pain. These may be used in conjunction with applying heat or ice (whichever you find more soothing) for 20 minutes to the neck and shoulders.

Three helpful techniques are described below:

- Oscillatory movements: small, rhythmic, side-to-side head movements, turning the head through about 25% of its full range of motion. Starting with your head facing forward, first turn your head away from the painful side and back. Repeat at a rate of about 1 per second, for a total of 30 seconds. Rest for 30 seconds; then repeat until no further relief is noted. Then switch to turning the head toward the painful side, and proceed as above.
- Positional distraction: Place books on the floor in a stack that is about 1–2 inches high. Lie down on the floor, with the back of your head resting on the books. The edge of the books should be near the middle of your head, so that your neck is free. Relax so that your head moves up from your neck.
- Trigger-point compression: during a headache, you may notice certain spots on your muscles that aggravate the head pain when you press them. These are called trigger points. If you identify trigger points, apply pressure to them with your fingers and hold for 12–60 seconds. Release the pressure, and proceed with your usual stretching exercises.

Nausea Treatment

What can I do if I'm feeling nauseated during my pregnancy?

- Fluids will be better tolerated if they are cold, clear, and carbonated, and consumed in small amounts between meals. Options include ginger ale or lemon-lime soda, clear broth, juice diluted with water, gelatin, electrolyte drinks (e.g., Gatorade and Pedialyte), and popsicles.
- When nausea has improved, move on to the "BRAT" diet: **B**ananas, **R**ice, **A**pplesauce, and **T**oast. Eat only small portions.
- Choose salty over sweet foods.
- Avoid hot, spicy, fried, greasy, or high-fat food.
- If food odors make you nauseated, use prepared or frozen foods or let someone else do the cooking. Another trick is to use a nose clip to minimize the odors.
- Eat in a cool, well-ventilated room, away from where the food was prepared.
- Eat slowly.
- Supplements containing iron can increase nausea and may need to be temporarily reduced.
- An empty stomach may aggravate nausea, so eat snacks frequently and as soon as you feel hungry.
- Keep dry crackers by your bedside. Eat a few crackers in the morning before rising and then sit upright in bed for a few minutes before getting up. This will often minimize the feeling of nausea that occurs with an empty stomach.

Additional Headache Resources

Where can I find reliable online information about migraine and other headaches?

Some of the best sites for getting reliable and up-to-date information on migraine and other headaches are managed by national headache foundations:

- American Council for Headache Education at http://www.achenet.org
- American Headache Society at http://www.ahsnet.org/resources/patient.php
- National Headache Foundation at http://www.headaches.org

These sites provide information on testing, diaries, diets, and treatment, as well as specialized topics like migraines in kids, pregnant women, and people with fibromyalgia.

The following sites provide specific information about the safety of medications during pregnancy and breastfeeding:

- The Hospital for Sick Children of the University of Toronto at http://www.motherisk.com
- King's College London at http://www.safefetus.com/
- Thomas W. Hale, RPh, PhD, Professor of Pediatrics at Texas Tech University at http://neonatal.ttuhsc.edu/lact/

Where can I learn more about managing headaches?

There are many excellent books that describe effective ways to manage your headache. You may wish to take advantage of information in some of the books listed below:

- **General information**
  - Bernstein C, McArdle E. 2008. *The migraine brain. Your breakthrough guide to fewer headaches, better health.* Glencoe, IL: Free Press.
  - Foster CA. 2007. *Migraine. Your questions answered.* New York, NY: DK Publishing.
  - Roberts T. 2005. *Living well with migraine disease and headaches: You're your doctor doesn't tell you ... that you need to know.* New York, NY: Harper Collins.
  - Kenefick K. 2006. *Migraines be gone: 7 simple steps to eliminating your migraines forever.* Crestone, CO: Roots and Wings Publishing.
  - Marcus DA. 2006. *10 simple solutions to migraine.* Oakland, CA: New Harbinger.
  - Blumenthal M, Brinckmann J, Wollschlaeger B. 2003. *The ABC clinical guide to herbs.* New York, NY: Thieme.

- **Safety of medications and supplements during pregnancy and nursing**
  - Briggs GG, Freeman RK, Yaffe SJ. 2008. *Drugs in pregnancy and lactation: a reference guide to fetal and neonatal risk, 8th edition.* Portland, OR: Lippincott Williams & Wilkins.
  - Hale TW. 2008. *Medications and mothers' milk: a manual of lactational pharmacology.* Amarillo, TX: Pharmasoft Medical Publishing.
  - Humphrey S. 2003. *The nursing mother's herbal.* Fairview Press.
  - Rubin SH. 2008. *The ABCs of breastfeeding: everything a mom needs to know for a happy nursing experience.* New York, NY: AMACOM.

- **Guides to learning non-drug treatments**
  - Davis M, Eshelman ER, McKay M. 2000. *The relaxation & stress reduction workbook.* Oakland, CA: Raincoast Books.
  - Delaune V. 2008. *Trigger point therapy for headaches & migraines: your self-treatment workbook for pain relief.* Oakland, CA: Raincoast Books.
  - Rossman M. *Headache relief: guided imagery exercises to soothe, relax and heal (guided self-healing practices).* Sounds True, 2004. [Audio CD]
  - Sharpe M. 2001. *The migraine cookbook: more than 100 healthy and delicious recipes for migraine sufferers.* New York, NY: Marlowe & Co.
  - Magee E. 2005. *Tell me what to eat if I have headaches and migraine.* Franklin Lakes, NJ: The Career Press.

- Van Houten P. 2003. *Yoga therapy for headache relief.* Nevada City, CA: Crystal Clarity Publishers.

• **Helping your child with headaches**
  - Zeltzer LK, Schlank CB. 2005. *Conquering your child's chronic pain: a pediatrician's guide for reclaiming a normal childhood.* New York, NY: HarperCollins.
  - Diamond S, Diamond A. 2001. *Headache and your child: the complete guide to understanding and treating migraine and other headaches in children and adolescents.* New York, NY: Fireside.
  - Culbert T, Kajander R. 2007. *Be the boss of your pain: self-care for kids.* Minneapolis, MN: Free Spirit Publishing.
  - Ricker J. 2006. *The headache detective: mom, my head hurts.* Massillon, OH: Thomas and Clayton Publishing.

Index

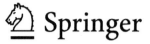

Printed in the United States of America